W9-BBG-613

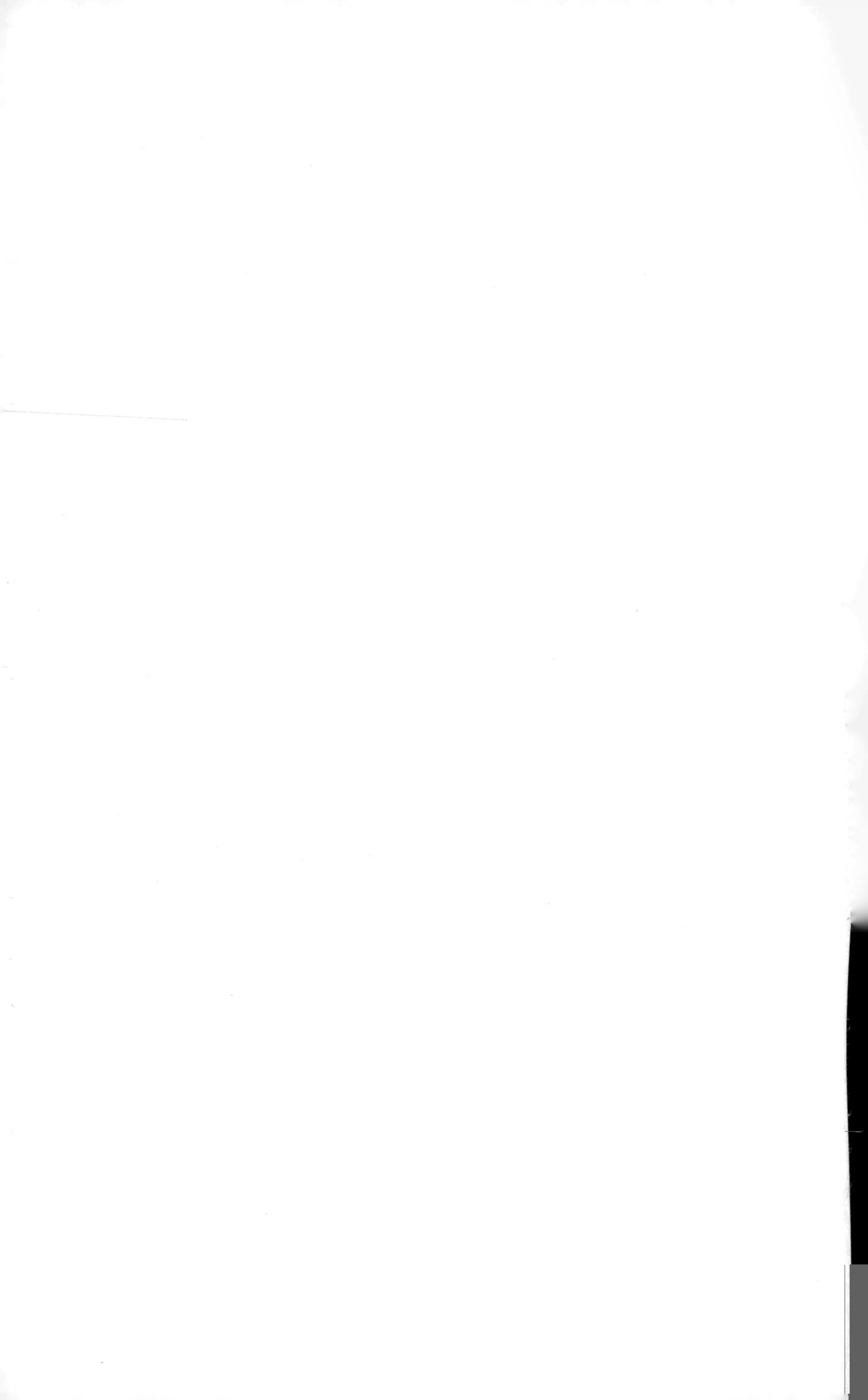

SCARLET A

SCARLET A

The Ethics, Law, and Politics of Ordinary Abortion

Katie Watson

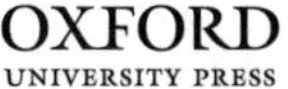
OXFORD UNIVERSITY PRESS

OXFORD
UNIVERSITY PRESS

Oxford University Press is a department of the University of Oxford. It furthers the University's objective of excellence in research, scholarship, and education by publishing worldwide. Oxford is a registered trade mark of Oxford University Press in the UK and certain other countries.

Published in the United States of America by Oxford University Press
198 Madison Avenue, New York, NY 10016, United States of America.

CIP data is on file at the Library of Congress
ISBN 978–0–19–062485–9

1 3 5 7 9 8 6 4 2

Printed by Sheridan Books, Inc., United States of America

For the mother and father who made me, and the husband and son who sustain me. The luck of having you is astounding.

CONTENTS

SCARLET A

Introduction

It caught my eye after I left the Vatican. An imposing medieval building loomed over the riverbank, and sticking out of its wall was an odd little stone box with a tiny roof on it. Was it a wishing well? I walked closer and saw the box had an open front, and it contained half of a wooden barrel. The barrel was cut top-to-bottom with a pole in the center. I touched it, and the half-barrel spun. What was this peculiar thing?

My tourist's guide to Rome told me I was at Santo Spirito Hospital, and what I was turning between the exterior and interior of the hospital was the first "foundling wheel"—a place parents could set an unwanted baby, rotate it into the hospital, then run down the street and around the corner before a nun could reach the hospital's front door and identify them. Pope Innocent III ordered its installation around the year 1200 because people sometimes drowned their unwanted babies in the Tiber River. Foundling Wheels offered a new response to unwanted pregnancy: the ability to anonymously leave a baby to be raised by strangers. Spinning that eight-hundred-year-old wheel reminded me what an old question *Roe v. Wade* revolved around: "I'm pregnant, but I don't want to have a baby. What can I do?"

Today's discussion of that question in the United States includes the option of safe abortion. Abortion has long existed in methods such as toxic herbs that sometimes induced miscarriage. "Safe abortion" is a new category. Reliably safe and effective abortion became a medical option in the 1900s after advances in surgical and antiseptic techniques. It became a legal option in the United States in the late 1960s when some states decriminalized it, and in 1973 nationally when the U.S. Supreme Court addressed it.*

"Surgical abortion" was the first type of safe abortion—procedures that end pregnancy by putting medical instruments inside the uterus. Today the most common method of surgical abortion is vacuum aspiration (suction), which can end a first-trimester pregnancy in five minutes. In 2000, a second type of safe abortion became legal in the United States—"medical abortion" uses FDA-approved pills (often called "the abortion pill") that trigger miscarriage of an embryo if taken up to 10 weeks after the first day of the last menstrual period. The procedures and pharmaceuticals that collectively constitute "safe abortion" are rarely discussed as a new medical technology, but that's what they are. Together, these forms of safe, legal abortion mean that today the risk of dying from abortion in the United States is comparable to the risk of dying from a dental procedure.

Advances in medicine's ability to alter nature's path regularly raise contentious questions. Our creation of technology like ventilators

* "Safe" and "legal" are different categories. For example, when abortion was illegal in the United States, some physicians clandestinely performed safe abortions in their offices, and a group of women in Chicago called "Jane" performed over ten thousand safe abortions through their underground service. In our era of legal abortion, some women still try unsafe abortion methods at home, and rogue doctor Kermit Gosnell was recently convicted of killing one abortion patient and injuring others. But legality dramatically improves abortion's safety. Legality allowed almost all abortions in the United States to move to medical professionals working in licensed medical facilities, and it allowed those professionals to receive specialized training, and to openly conduct and share the medical research that developed new procedures with even less risk. Legality also helps women end unwanted pregnancies earlier by allowing open access to information about where one can find an abortion provider, which makes abortion safer overall since delay increases risk.

forces us to confront questions about when life ends, and our creation of safe abortion forces us to confront questions about when life begins. Is abortion late birth control? Early infanticide? Or something in between?

In *Roe v. Wade* (1973), the U.S. Supreme Court ruled that the Constitution doesn't give government the power to answer those questions. Instead, before viability (the point at which a fetus might be able to survive outside the womb), that power lies with individual citizens and their doctors, who must be allowed to follow their individual conscience and religious beliefs in answering those questions for themselves.

"Liberty finds no refuge in a jurisprudence of doubt," Justice Sandra Day O'Connor wrote in *Casey v. Pennsylvania*, the 1992 case that affirmed *Roe*'s holding that abortion is a constitutional right. In other words, citizens deserve the kind of clarity and stability in constitutional law that allows them to move forward with their lives. But in the twenty-six years since *Casey*, the incessant battle over abortion has created some of the doubt Justice O'Connor hoped would be eliminated by explicitly affirming *Roe*.

When those who want abortion outlawed weren't successful in the Supreme Court, they adopted a new strategy: pass state laws making this constitutionally protected right difficult or impossible to exercise. In addition to erecting barriers, this flood of abortion regulation has created confusion. I'm a bioethics professor at a medical school, and the fact that quite a few of my incredibly smart medical students begin their training unclear if and when abortion is legal concerns me. For people who do know the law, the fact that legislatures keep passing these regulations, and courts often allow them, creates an accurate impression that the abortion right is under siege, and a legitimate fear that *Roe* could be reversed someday. So although abortion has been legal across the United States for forty-five years, we act as if it could become illegal any day now.

But the sky hasn't fallen yet. The basic right that the Supreme Court acknowledged in 1973 and affirmed in 1992—that abortion is a matter of individual conscience before viability—hasn't been openly addressed by the Supreme Court since, and in 2016 the Court wrote as if the abortion right was a given in the case of *Whole Woman's Health v. Hellerstedt*. So in this book I write as if abortion is legal in the United States, because it is.

In addition to being a bioethicist I'm a lawyer, but I've resisted my lawyerly impulse to write yet another constitutional law book rearguing *Roe* and I've dropped the legalese. I explain some of the reasons abortion is constitutionally protected, and why *Roe* should be considered settled law that America accepts. But my larger goal is to set that aside, because our focus on the Supreme Court, and our feelings of uncertainty and anxiety about the law, have paralyzed another part of the abortion conversation.

In a country where abortion has been a constitutional right for forty-five years, we should be able to move on to a richer conversation about ethics and morality. We should be able to acknowledge the complexity of private decisionmaking without threatening the *right* of private decisionmaking. I'm worried about what the divisiveness of abortion politics is doing to our country, and I don't think much legal compromise is possible or desirable. Instead, I think good things would happen if we shifted our collective focus away from the public sphere of law, and toward the private conversations in which ordinary people decide whether or not to exercise the rights the Constitution protects.

Yet it's hard to talk about abortion. The public conversation feels toxic, and I fear a desire to avoid its corrosive polarization has shut down private conversation. Which is a problem, because that's how people usually work things out—in private, sincere exchanges of experience and opinion to which neither person has brought a bullhorn. I also sense a collective exhaustion, and sometimes boredom, with the topic. Professors tell me you can't teach a class on abortion; senior ethicists have told me there's nothing new to say. The abortion stories on the news sound repetitive and abortion politics can be vicious. So if you don't think you or anyone you know is affected by abortion, why bother? And if you or someone you know is affected by abortion, why wouldn't you keep it to yourself?

In this book I will first suggest that abortion might be more relevant to you than you realize. And if it's been directly relevant to you, I'll suggest there are good reasons to let a few more people know that. Approximately 3 out of 10 American women who are currently age 45 or older have had one or more abortions. Looking forward, approximately 1 in 4 American women who are currently 44 years old or younger are expected to have one or more in the future.*

Why isn't something this common discussed in ordinary day-to-day conversation? Because abortion is our era's Scarlet A.

In *The Scarlet Letter*, Hester Prynne's pregnancy reveals that she committed the sin of adultery, and her Puritan community sentences her to forever wear a scarlet A as a sign of shame. Stigma is an invisible mark of shame or social disgrace that triggers a response like the letter on Hester's dress. Today, abortion stigma brands the women and couples who have them and the health care professionals who provide them with an invisible scarlet A. To keep everyone else from seeing it, most of them hide their A. Something such a large number of American women decide to do (in conjunction with their male partners, in a majority of cases) is not a fringe practice. But our silence on the topic leads even those who do it to believe otherwise.

* The estimate has changed from 1-in-3 to 1-in-4 because abortion rates are going down, a trend I discuss later in this book. "Lifetime incidence" of abortion is a helpful concept, and a bit of a moving target. It was estimated to be 43% in 1992, then in 2008 it dropped to 30%. Data that will be published around the time this book goes to press show that if 2014 rates prevail, 24% of American women who were 15–44 that year will have an abortion in their lifetime.

One result of our public and private silence about the experience of abortion is that doctors and clinic managers have become the public face of abortion. Unlike other health issues, in which patients and families advocate for future patients and the doctors and institutions that helped them, in abortion we ask those who provide something millions of women and families want and need to also shoulder most of the burden of its defense. That doesn't seem fair, and I don't think it's sustainable.

The missing topic of conversation is what I call ordinary abortion. The advocates who drive the public abortion discussion often highlight what I think of as extraordinary abortion—extreme cases of abortion need, and extreme cases of what opponents might call "abortion abuse." Those supporting its legality tend to highlight cases of rape, terrible fetal anomaly, and pregnant twelve-year-olds. Those opposing its legality often highlight "late abortion," advancing bans on abortion in the second trimester, and bans on a second-trimester procedure they framed as partial birth abortion.

To observe that advocates tend to focus on extraordinary abortion is not a criticism of either side—it makes rhetorical sense to focus on the cases that evoke the strongest emotions. Focusing public debate on extremes also has the benefit of keeping it comfortable for the many Americans who care about women *and* embryos or fetuses. Cases that create intense empathy for one side of the equation nearly erase the other, and that allows us to avoid our ambivalence. The focus on extraordinary abortion is reinforced by the media. In addition to reporting on extreme cases and extreme political clashes, the news tells us about extraordinary abortion opposition (such as the 2015 shootings at a Planned Parenthood in Colorado) or particularly large protests. Again, this is not a criticism—the imperatives of reporting preclude this headline: "Peaceful day at abortion clinic: ordinary people got quality healthcare." Peaceful days of quality care happen much more than shootings and protests, but the ordinary is the antithesis of news. The absence of the ordinary in our public abortion conversation fuels an image of abortion as constantly embattled. Abortion *is* embattled, but that's only part of the picture.

The absence of the ordinary means the cases we discuss most are the ones that occur least. Most of the extraordinary cases of American abortion that advocates and the media offer really happen. They are important, and calling them extraordinary is not meant to marginalize or minimize them. Discussing them can clarify our thinking, and that's why I occasionally mention this kind of extraordinary case too. And numerically, since women in the United States have approximately one million abortions a year, a "type" that is 1% of abortion experience is still 10,000 cases. But statistically, extraordinary abortion is a small minority of abortion experiences. I think it's odd that our public discourse doesn't reflect the majority of private experiences. In this book I consider why this disjuncture exists, what it might cost us, and what might be gained by talking about the cases that represent the majority of patient and provider experiences. Ordinary abortion.

Talking about any kind of abortion tests our tolerance for ambiguity, because the relationship between pregnant women and their embryos or fetuses is so unlike other relationships, and embryos and fetuses are so unlike other individuals. Ambiguity leads to distress, and that leads a lot of people to decide it's easier to not talk about abortion at all. But I think this conversation is too important to walk away from.

This book is for anyone who is sick of the anti-woman, anti-sex, political pot-stirring motivations for talking about the morality of abortion. It's for people who are unresolved but have dropped out of the abortion conversation because a shrill tone has made it feel unpleasant or unproductive. And it's for people who feel resolved about their own position (whether pro or con) but feel unable to talk to people who see things differently.

A discussion of abortion ethics that's premised on legality also opens space for two groups our polarizing public debates may have pushed out. I think of the first group as pro-choice/anti-abortion: Americans who think abortion should remain legal, but who have deep ethical concerns about the practice. This book is intended to engage ambivalent pro-choice people who would like to move the conversation from "can you" to "should you." The second group is on the opposite end of the ethics spectrum—Americans who think of abortion not as a "necessary evil" (a bad thing we must allow), but instead as morally good. Our current political climate makes it virtually impossible for anyone to consider themselves "pro-abortion." But the perspectives of people who do not think the destruction of embryonic life is a significant moral problem, and who think the freedom abortion gives women is a significant moral good, are valuable in this conversation as well.

I began this research because I wanted to clarify my own thinking and talking about abortion. This book reflects a journey I've taken as a professor of bioethics and medical humanities, a lawyer, a woman, and now a mother. In one phase of this book's gestation I was also pregnant, and experiencing everything from early nausea triggered by an embryo, the kickboxing of a third-trimester fetus, childbirth, and nurturing a newborn made the topics I was writing about even more visceral.

I am not a philosopher, a social scientist, an English professor, a doctor, or a scientist, although I draw from all those fields. I am also not an abortion scholar; those who are will see many omissions here from a rich literature too vast to capture in one book. I'm a bioethicist who noticed something funny: that the frequency of patients asking doctors to perform a particular medical intervention (abortion) didn't seem to be part of the larger conversation about that area of medicine (abortion care). Later I noticed that the amount of attention this medical specialty got from society far outweighed the attention it got from bioethicists, which seemed odd to me as well.

Bioethics is a multidisciplinary field that contains scholars from all the fields noted above and then some. My home discipline is law, and later I was trained in clinical medical ethics. My background in professional roles that required me to make recommendations may explain why I don't pretend to be undecided. Some academic authors refrain from offering their own conclusions to maintain an appearance of objectivity. I think it's more useful to say openly that my analysis has led me to a pro-choice position. But the fact I've reached a conclusion (which doesn't distinguish me from many, so perhaps I should say the fact I *disclose* the conclusion I've reached) doesn't mean I'm writing as an advocate. I am writing as an academic, which means I work hard to be honest in my data selection, fair in my analysis, and transparent in my reasoning. My agenda is to improve the American abortion debate and my hope is that all readers, those who disagree with me as well as those who agree, will be able to use my work to clarify and strengthen their own reasoning and conclusions, so we can continue the conversation together.

In Chapter 1 I begin with something that isn't usually included in the abortion debate: the voting we do with our feet, as opposed to ballots or opinion polls. The legal and political circus of American abortion policy and the stigma-triggered silence of patients have made it easy to miss that millions are quietly using this service. Yet one prerequisite of productive conversation is knowing what's currently happening. Philosophical treatises on abortion deal in abstractions, but in real-life moral reasoning we're always integrating ideas with experience. So I start with the practice of abortion before moving to the idea of abortion. Throughout the book I illustrate statistics with stories of real women and men—patients, physicians, and others—who either shared their abortion experiences with me in interviews, or published their own accounts.

In Chapters 2 and 3 I explore abortion narrative and vocabulary, because another prerequisite of productive conversation is the thoughtful use of language. Words and stories don't just express our thinking, they help shape it. I use judicial opinions as my texts, to give those unfamiliar with abortion law a primer, and those who are familiar with the law a different way to think about it. First I consider storytelling, because expanding the types of abortion stories and opinions people feel free to share, and the range of them we are truly able to hear, will help us better understand the full range of experience in this area. Then I focus on vocabulary, illustrating why it's so hard to construct a "neutral" sentence about abortion, and offering best alternatives. The public abortion debate reduces life's complexity to black and white. My hope is that insights and tools that help us have nuanced private conversation will spark a shift toward civility and depth in our public abortion conversations as well.

In Chapters 4 and 5 I explore abortion ethics—whether abortion is ever ethical, and if so, when. To say the U.S. Constitution gives women the right to end an unwanted pregnancy is only the beginning of a conversation. Yet the toxicity of our national conflict over abortion law has made honest discussion of abortion ethics seem impossible. These chapters assume abortion's legality so we can move the conversation forward from "rights" (which I think must be preserved) to "the right thing to do" (which the law leaves up to you). Women and couples facing unintended pregnancy are split—42% abort, and 58% continue the pregnancy. Given the right to continue or end an unwanted pregnancy, how could or should people decide whether to exercise this right? Which of the many approaches to abortion ethics I review best captures your perspective? The primary focus of these chapters is on the private decision-making and personal opinion that flourish in a pluralistic society. However, to illustrate how these ethics theories play out in the public sphere I also identify statutes and judicial decisions consistent with each one.

In Chapter 6 I consider the politics of abortion—not the constant battles in the legislatures and courts, but the deeper structural, cultural, and social issues that help fuel these fires. First I consider the

"Trojan Horse" problem, and how state regulations that falsely purport to protect women's health create structural stigma. Then I consider the "Russian Doll" problem, in which debates about the moral status of embryos and fetuses hide other debates we're not having openly (but should) on topics like gender roles, sexuality, and religion. I end on issues of Realpolitik—how might we move the public conversation forward?

Women face many forms of reproductive injustice besides the stigma and barriers that surround ending an unwanted pregnancy. This book focuses on abortion because access to the service is threatened and misunderstood. However, my focus on abortion is not intended to suggest that other issues vital to the larger framework of reproductive justice—such as access to contraception, access to medically accurate reproductive education, access to culturally competent care, access to assisted reproductive technology, freedom from domestic violence, freedom from the poverty that prevents women from continuing wanted pregnancies, access to affordable high-quality childcare, the forced medical treatment of pregnant women, the criminal prosecution of pregnant women, and the right to parent—are not pressing. They are, particularly for women of color, low-income women, and immigrant women, and all these issues deserve a depth of analysis that is beyond the scope of this book.

When I was in Rome spinning the Foundling Wheel of Santo Spirito Hospital, I was moved by the thought of every woman who had stood there before me, entering a darkened street a half-mile from the Sistine Chapel, about to let go of her baby. Because she and her husband couldn't afford to feed one more child? Because the stigma of an illegitimate child would ruin her? Running my fingers along the barrel's rough wood I wondered what these women felt in this moment. Grief? Relief? A complex constellation of emotions as unique as each woman herself? Then they sprinted down the stone street into the night, before anyone could see their faces.

Roe v. Wade didn't start our country's conflict. How individuals and societies should respond to unwanted pregnancy is a very old question. When a question has remained contentious across centuries, perhaps rather than seeing it as a problem to be solved, it's more helpful to think of it as one of the ongoing struggles of life.

This book isn't a blueprint for a new conversation. It's an explanation of why we need one, and an invitation to participate in moving that forward.

A Note on Terminology

Issues of language are discussed throughout this book, but the term "pro-life" should be considered at the outset. Many physicians and nurses who provide abortion care are insulted by this term's implicit "anti-life" accusation. These medical professionals argue that they are passionately "pro-life," because abortion's legalization all but eliminated American women's chance of being killed or injured by the procedure, and their desire to save women's lives is why they do this difficult work. The murder and injury of their colleagues by extremists claiming the "pro-life" mantle only increases its sting. I respect the mainstream on both sides of this issue and believe both care about "life." Therefore, I use the term "pro-life" to describe a view that abortion should be illegal only when I'm paraphrasing someone else's views, or when clarity requires it. When the shorthand for positions is up to me, I avoid the term.

What's a fair alternative to "pro-life"? "Anti-choice" is factually accurate (since those who want to make abortion illegal or impossible seek to eliminate the only alternative to childbirth a pregnant person has), but pro-choice/anti-choice is an unfair mismatch in spirit because everyone's *for* something. So in my own analysis I juxtapose pro-choice with "pro-fetal rights." That is an accurate summary of this position's core argument—an embryo or fetus should have legal rights that sometimes or always trump the rights of the woman carrying it. And the fact that pro-choice and pro-fetal rights are both legal positions helps clarify whether we're discussing law or ethics, a clarity of topic I argue is required for productive conversation. I describe the position of a person who thinks abortion should remain legal, and also thinks it is an unethical or immoral act that people shouldn't do, as "pro-choice/anti-abortion." (It could also be called "pro-choice/pro-embryonic and fetal life.")

I know these terms will be unsatisfactory to some who describe themselves as pro-life. For example, a law and bioethics professor I like and respect has a position that's hard to capture with simple labels. She identifies as pro-life, but for her that means much more than "anti-abortion." Her use of the term is grounded in Cardinal Bernardin's "seamless garment" philosophy of respect for the dignity of all life, meaning she also opposes war and the death penalty, and advocates for immigrants and those in poverty. She's a feminist who opposes almost all the current restrictions states have placed on abortion because she thinks they demean women and their difficult decisions. In her estimation, these state laws seem to care very little for taking care of women, pregnant women, children, and families, so she sees them as anti-abortion rather than truly pro-life. However, she does not support laws that allow abortion. She would prefer to see abortion decriminalized rather than legalized, meaning it would be illegal, but sanctioned only with fines or civil penalties that are perhaps not even enforced. Given the current political climate, her focus at a pragmatic and ethical level is reducing the reasons that women choose abortion. I asked her opinion on my "pro-choice/anti-abortion" label and she quickly rejected it. She doesn't want to relinquish the breadth she sees in the term "pro-life," and she doesn't want to adopt the political connotations of the term "pro-choice." To readers like her and all others with complex views on this sensitive topic, let me acknowledge the limits of language, and invite you to substitute the terms you prefer as you read.

Pseudonyms

In this book, I have used the real names of those who I quote from publications they've written. I offered everyone I spoke with the option of a pseudonym, and use one whenever that was her or his preference. A list of these is as follows:

Amelia Danforth
Dr. Catherine Tate
Paul
Martha Ashe
Kara Evans, APN
Betty
Dr. Penelope Lasalle
Midwestern Hospital
Christopher Lapin

Chapter 1

Ordinary Abortion

Common and Clandestine

Amelia Danforth was thrilled to be living her dream, finally supporting herself as an actor in a touring production of a play, when she got pregnant the first time she slept with Mike. Amelia is a petite, freckly brunette who shares many details of her life with a large circle of loving friends and family. But after she and Mike had an abortion, she only told one friend. Why did she treat her abortion so differently from the rest of her love life and health news? "There's never a good time to tell your abortion story," Amelia told me. "At what dinner party is it a good time?"

Amelia is not alone. Many women have abortions, and many women keep quiet about it. According to the latest data, one in five American pregnancies ends in abortion (19%). Did you know that?

I didn't. Then I was assigned to teach a medical school class on reproductive ethics. I researched abortion's frequency, and I was shocked. I thought the statistics couldn't be right. Medically, miscarriage is called "spontaneous abortion," and when an embryo or fetus doesn't pass from the body naturally after miscarriage, people have abortions to avoid infection. "Aha!" I thought. "The idea that 3 out of 10 women have an abortion must include miscarriages where the medical procedure is called 'abortion,' but because the embryo or fetus died before the procedure, the rest of us don't think of it that way." Nope—I checked and the statistics include only "ongoing pregnancies." My students were amazed too. And this was in medical school. Why didn't we all know this?

Because abortion is our era's Scarlet A. Amelia puts it this way: "Every once in a while I'm sitting in a room full of my family and my friends, and something comes up and I think, 'I could talk about my abortion now, we're all adults.' And it's like, no you can't! This isn't a thing you can bring up." Why not? Does she feel ashamed of it? "No. It feels combative to bring it up. Which is weird! Like in one way I'd be trying to incite someone, and in another way to make someone feel bad for me ... [and] I don't want either of those things."

Talking to Amelia made me think back to an exchange I had many years ago. I was getting a haircut, and as I sat in the salon chair I complained to my hairdresser's reflection in the mirror that my hair had yo-yo'd between straight and curly over the years.

"It's usually hormones," my upbeat new hairdresser said. "Have you ever been pregnant?"

"No."

She leaned closer to the mirror. "Abortions count!"

I laughed, startled. "Yeah. No. I haven't been pregnant."

"Hmm," she replied, raising her scissors to tackle my mysterious mess.

This hardly qualifies as an abortion story, but it stands out to me as the only time I've heard the possibility of an abortion acknowledged in a routine conversation. In contemporary American culture, people often share a vast range of personal detail about life events and medical procedures—just not abortion. So while politicians and pundits yell about abortion, ordinary people keep pretty quiet. My hairdresser's friendly, transgressive "abortions count!" amused me at the time, but after I learned about the way abortion stigma generates silence, I admired the matter-of-fact way she raised the possibility—just a nonjudgmental clinician trying to diagnose my hair. But Amelia is right. Talking about her abortion at a dinner party would be shocking.

American abortion is both common and clandestine. These elements combine to create what scholars call "the prevalence paradox." Many women in the United States have abortions. Yet because abortion is stigmatized, even people who describe themselves as pro-choice, like Amelia, don't want to be associated with it. The silence surrounding abortion makes it seem uncommon, perpetuating a social norm that abortion is deviant even though statistically it's common. Stigma produces silence, silence produces stigma, and this circular effect produces the prevalence paradox. People keep quiet about their association with abortion to avoid the discrimination imposed on deviants, and something many people do continues to be misperceived as uncommon.

Learning about abortion's frequency changed how I think about it, and my quest to understand the prevalence paradox is part of what motivated this book. In the United States, over 30 million women have had legal abortions since *Roe v. Wade* was decided in 1973. To make sense of that number, picture it this way: if all these women came together on the 45th anniversary of *Roe* in 2018, they would replace the population of the entire states of Texas, Nevada, and Maine. Put another way, if all the women who ended pregnancies with legal abortion services between 1973 and 2014 were still living, they would be 25% of adult women in the United States.

Numbers like these made me feel there's something unreal about the American abortion conversation. Abortion's prevalence is rarely captured in personal conversation, political debates, or academic articles on the moral status of the fetus. Stigma means we hear more about the *idea* of abortion than the actual practice of abortion. But I think it's essential to discuss America's decades of abortion experience too. Then we can consider how practice should influence our ideas, and how ideas should influence our practice.

Acknowledging the prevalence of abortion in America opens the door to discussion of what I call "ordinary abortion." Calling the majority of the approximately one million abortions Americans have each year "ordinary" is not meant to diminish the significance abortion has to many. Some would say the intentional killing of an embryo or fetus can never be considered ordinary. Others would say a woman taking control of her body and life in defiance of cultural expectations of motherhood can never be considered ordinary.

I call these cases ordinary because they are the most common types of abortion. Ordinary abortion is the 74% of women ending pregnancies who say having a baby would dramatically change their life, interfering with work, school, or their ability to care for dependents; the 48% who say they don't want to be a single parent or they are having problems with their husband or partner; the 73% who say they cannot afford a child.* I call them ordinary because they happen frequently—these cases are the majority of the approximately 55 million abortions American women chose to have between 1973 and 2014.

These abortions are also ordinary medically. Practically speaking, they are safe, routine medical procedures. Conceptually speaking, they are consistent with the goals of medicine: at a patient's request, a physician brings the patient's body back to its baseline state. Pregnancy is not an injury or an illness, and abortion decisionmaking is different from other medical decisionmaking because it includes whatever moral weight the woman or couple and the physician assign

* These numbers add to more than 100 because patients could check more than one reason. Of the 13 reasons offered, the median number of reasons women gave was four. When asked the most important reason for having the abortion, 25% selected "Not ready for another child/timing is wrong," 23% selected "Can't afford a baby now," and 19% selected "Have completed my childbearing/have other people depending on me/children are grown."

the embryo or fetus. But in the United States, where the average woman currently has 2 children over the course of a seventy-plus-year lifespan, the baseline status of an American woman's body is to not be pregnant. Whether a patient is unhappy about a broken leg, a lung infection, or an unwanted pregnancy, in ordinary medicine a patient tells a doctor he or she doesn't want the health risks and life-altering effects of a change in his or her body, and the doctor uses a drug or procedure to bring the body back to the way it was.

To say something is common or routine is not to say that it's good. But acknowledging the prevalence of American abortion raises a question of moral intuition.

Tens of millions of Americans have voted with their feet over the course of forty-five years to say the moral status of embryos, fetuses, and women permits abortion. Is it possible that many millions of Americans are all depraved or misguided? "Everyone's doing it" is not a winning ethical argument. But it is a piece of evidence that deserves serious consideration. In Chapters 4 and 5 I review a range of philosophical arguments about the moral status of embryos and fetuses, some of which maintain all these people have done a terrible thing. For now I simply observe that decades of pro-life arguments haven't persuaded over 30 million patients and many of their partners. The patients' rights and medical ethics revolutions of the 1970s were premised on the idea that ordinary people were serious moral thinkers who were entitled to request or refuse medical care according to their own values. I see no reason to grant any lesser status to the women and couples who decide abortion is right for them.

While advocates argue about rights, politicians cozy up to interest groups, and scholars analyze abstractions, Americans' behavior has quietly established abortion as routine medical care. Discussion of American abortion often includes opinion polling, and people's opinions about abortion are important. But only looking at polls is like the mistake of guarding a basketball player by focusing on her head. If you only watch where her eyes tell you she's going, she can fool you. Follow where her chest says she's going instead. Follow the body.

Dr. Catherine Tate is an obstetrician/gynecologist who wears her curly blond hair gathered in a loose bun and looks like a grad student in the sweatshirt and jeans she favors when she's not at work. When she's seeing patients at an abortion clinic, she asks her staff to flag any patients who seem distraught so she can talk to them personally before they go on to the next standard step of meeting with the clinic's counselor. One day the staff told her a patient was unusually tearful during her sonogram and seemed angry at the sonographer. Dr. Tate went to the patient's room to learn more and was startled to recognize the pregnant woman on this urban abortion clinic's exam table. She was an anti-abortion protester Dr. Tate had recently seen picketing at a college town's clinic two hours away. (A clinic merger had led Dr. Tate to cover shifts in the college town's clinic five or six times in a four- or five-month period, and Dr. Tate had seen the woman picketing on all of those days.)

"Are you sure this is the best decision for you today?" Dr. Tate asked. The patient, a white woman in her early 30s dressed like a white-collar professional, told Dr. Tate abortion is terrible and should be illegal, because if abortion were illegal, she wouldn't be doing this. "But I'm weak," she told Dr. Tate, "so because it's legal I'm here doing the wrong thing." The woman had filled out paperwork saying she'd had one previous abortion, but her picketing led Dr. Tate to surmise she'd changed her beliefs since then, so she probed further: "I feel like I recognize you from seeing you outside our other clinic location. Is that right?" The patient was surprised—she hadn't recognized Dr. Tate—but seemed unfazed. "Yes. Abortion is ending a life, it's never the right option. But this is what I need to do."

Cases like that of Dr. Tate's patient remind me that it's important to consider both behavior and belief in the American abortion discussion. Abortion begins with opinion, but ultimately it's about action. What we do and say are different things—sometimes they're in sync, sometimes they aren't. That's true in many areas of life, and abortion is no exception. I don't mean to suggest that everyone with anti-abortion beliefs secretly behaves differently, but I'm struck by how many physicians and counselors have told me about patients requesting abortions who express strong opposition to abortion. The frequency with which abortion providers hear patients say "I'm against abortion but my case is different" leads some providers to joke that the conservative exceptions to abortion bans are "rape, incest, and me."

Some people see the "rape, incest, and me" philosophy in Scott DesJarlais, a pro-fetal rights congressman. He and his ex-wife Susan terminated two pregnancies while they were dating, then he urged another partner to terminate a pregnancy after he was married. Why? In his sworn testimony during divorce proceedings he explained the first was because Susan "was on an experimental drug called Lupron and was not supposed to have gotten pregnant. There were potential risks. It was a therapeutic [abortion]." The second "was after [Susan] had gotten back from Desert Storm and things were not going well between us and it was a mutual decision." Five years after marrying they separated and Representative DesJarlais, who is a physician, had a sexual relationship with a patient who later told him she was pregnant. He and Susan reconciled, and according to his testimony, together they recorded a phone call in which he urged this woman to have an abortion. In the transcript of the call he says he wants them to "get this solved and get it over with so we can get on with our lives...."

DesJarlais's reasons for wanting these three pregnancies to end in abortion—fear of fetal disability, relationship troubles, and a desire to prevent a brief sexual relationship from turning into a lifelong co-parenting relationship—are common. (As noted above, 48% of women obtaining abortions cite relationship problems. Thirteen percent cite possible problems affecting the health of the fetus.*) So after the Tennessee Republican benefited from safe, legal, accessible abortion, why does the "Issues" page of his official website say the following? "Abortion—Congressman DesJarlais believes that all life should be cherished and protected. He has received a 100% score by the National Right to Life Committee (NRLC), the oldest and the largest national pro-life organization in the United States."

Maybe Representative DesJarlais changed his beliefs over time. Or maybe it's simple hypocrisy—pretending to have beliefs you don't actually hold—designed to gain votes and power. Hypocrites and people who change their mind are two groups that are recognized in the abortion debate. A significant third group is rarely identified.

Some abortion patients and partners seem to be experiencing what psychologists call fundamental attribution error: the tendency to include circumstances (external factors) in explanations of our own behavior, but to blame other people's behavior on character (internal factors). If you're late to our meeting, I might think you're disrespectful or unorganized (character); if I'm late, it's because I'm juggling too many important obligations (circumstance). If kids in the news are on drugs, it's because they or their parents are derelicts; if my kid's on drugs, it's because she temporarily fell in with the wrong crowd.

At one level attribution error is understandable—I know every detail of my situation, and I don't know much about most other

* In the Endnotes to the Introduction supporting my definition of "extraordinary abortion," I said Guttmacher staff estimate that 1–2% of abortions are for fetal anomaly. That estimate for fetal anomalies diverges from the 13% of women reporting "possible problems affecting the health of the fetus" in the 2005 study because that survey item was not limited to fetal anomalies. Qualitative research suggests that women ending pregnancies use the term "health problems" to refer to their own exhaustion, their own pre-existing health conditions, fetal conditions they fear but which have not been diagnosed, or worries the embryo is damaged because they drank alcohol while pregnant. Jones RK, Frohwirth LF, Moore AM. "I would want to give my child, like, everything in the world": how issues of motherhood influence women who have abortions. *Journal of Family Issues*. Jan. 2008;29(1):79–99.

people's lives. It takes a generous spirit to imagine sympathetic circumstances motivating other people's behavior, especially when what they're doing upsets me. And the fact that we rarely hear about other people's abortion experiences only makes it harder to imagine why people other than ourselves come to an abortion clinic. Attribution error leads people in this third group to categorize abortions in their own lives differently from all other abortions: If I'm party to an accidental pregnancy that ends with abortion, it's because I/we/she made an honest mistake; when strangers end accidental pregnancies, it's because they're promiscuous, careless, or callous.

There are many reasons for the silence of patients like Amelia and others, but collectively that silence creates a hothouse in which fundamental attribution error can flourish. When Dr. Tate worked at a suburban clinic where the majority of patients were higher-income white women, "it seemed like many of them thought they didn't know anyone else who'd ever had an abortion—they thought they were the only one." The anti-abortion protester gave the same reasons for terminating a pregnancy that Dr. Tate hears from many patients, but "often the reasons that pulled-together white ladies come in with aren't nearly as extreme as others I hear. Yet I feel like they're more likely the ones who are judging others."

Dr. Tate was worried about the anti-abortion picketer who wanted to terminate her pregnancy. "It sounds like this isn't something you saw as part of your life, and I think you're at a high risk for regret," she told the patient. "What can we do to help you make sure you make the best decision for you today, including leaving here pregnant?" The patient said she couldn't have a baby with this man, she didn't want to be tied to him … that she couldn't be pregnant right now financially, where she was with her job … that she just couldn't be pregnant. Dr. Tate reminded the patient about the options of parenting or adoption, and suggested the patient go home and think about it. "Absolutely not," the patient insisted. Then the clinic social worker spoke to the patient, and this counselor confirmed what Dr. Tate heard—the patient never wavered from saying "this is what I want, this is what I need to do, this is the best decision for me." Dr. Tate was convinced that the anti-abortion protester sincerely wanted to end her pregnancy, and she decided it would be discriminatory to hold this patient to a higher standard than others. So she did what the protester asked.

About a month later, Dr. Tate went back to the college town for a day of work at that abortion clinic, and saw her patient again. The woman was back outside the clinic, carrying an anti-abortion sign. I wondered how Dr. Tate felt seeing her patient opposing the very service she had just requested and received for a second time. Was she tempted to "out" her, the way the same-sex lover of a politician who votes against gay rights might want to do? Dr. Tate seemed surprised by my question. "No. I felt like she's probably tormented enough. I don't need to add to that." So Dr. Tate honored doctor-patient confidentiality, walking past her former patient as if it were any other day.

But wasn't Dr. Tate angry? What was she thinking as she passed? Dr. Tate smiled. "Honestly? I thought, 'Looks like you recovered well. Good for safe and legal abortion.' "

The impact of safe and legal abortion goes beyond the women who choose to have one. I think of people like Congressman DesJarlais as "abortion beneficiaries"—people who didn't terminate a pregnancy themselves, but are glad someone else did.

Men who also didn't want to have a child are an obvious group that benefit from their partner's ability to choose a safe legal abortion, and I explore data on men and relationships further in Chapter 2. However, the web of abortion beneficiaries expands further than these men. For example, some people reading this book wouldn't exist if the abortion their mother had before they were born had been unsafe and robbed her of her fertility. Others wouldn't exist if their mother had continued that accidental pregnancy and, because she reached the maximum number of children she wanted to have, she used contraception that precluded them.

Every one of the approximately one million women who have a safe legal abortion each year is surrounded by people who benefited from the fact they didn't lose their beloved daughter, sister, mother, friend, or colleague to a deadly illegal abortion. Some parents who didn't have to raise a teenager's baby for her or him are abortion beneficiaries. Some people who had a better childhood than they would have had if another sibling had pushed their parents' income or energy past the breaking point are abortion beneficiaries.

The web of abortion beneficiaries even includes some people who aren't connected to a woman who's had one. (Although statistically, in the United States I'm not sure that's possible.) For example, all the unmarried and married couples who never had an accidental pregnancy, but have been able to enjoy their sex life because they weren't constantly afraid contraceptive failure would upend their lives, are beneficiaries. And some women and couples who become accidentally pregnant consider abortion before committing to parenthood, making their pregnancy experience and parenting relationship a product of their own affirmative choice rather than something the government forced on them.

An obvious response to the concept of "abortion beneficiary" is that abortion has robbed some people of a child, sibling, grandchild, colleague, etcetera, they would have loved to have had. (The moral status of embryos and fetuses is part of this calculus too. Few who think abortion is truly equivalent to murder would say their more comfortable childhood was worth a potential sibling's life; if you think abortion is nothing like murder, you might breathe a sigh of relief that you didn't go hungry.) That's why the concept of "abortion beneficiaries" is only meant to identify people who know about an abortion and feel they benefited from it, or don't know about the abortion but would feel they benefited from it if they learned it happened.

"Abortion culture" is meant as a derogatory description by those who oppose abortion. But honestly, they're on to something. Abortion has had a significant effect on a large number of Americans' lives. Safe legal abortion benefits many Americans who don't have the procedure themselves. It's impossible to quantify how many Americans are abortion beneficiaries, but together, they are all unrecognized stakeholders in the abortion debate.

The problem is that many people don't know they're abortion beneficiaries, because the mother, daughter, sister, friend, or colleague in their lives who had an abortion hasn't told them about it. In a study of over 4,000 women obtaining abortions at hospitals and clinics across the country, 58% of them agreed with the statement "I need to keep this abortion a secret from my close friends and family." (The study did not ask why women felt it must be kept secret.) Researchers call this internalized stigma. Forty percent agreed that "My friends and family would think less of me if they knew about this abortion," and 66% agreed "I would be looked down on by some people if they knew I'd had this abortion." Researchers call this perceived stigma. Of course this study can't say whether some of these women later disclosed their abortion to friends or family—and whether some who did were pleasantly surprised to learn they were wrong about the negative judgment they expected. (For example, in the decade that followed Amelia's abortion, she told three more friends about it and nothing bad happened.) But this study does document a high level of planned secrecy, and fear of judgment from the people who would usually form a woman's support network. The invisibility of abortion's Scarlet A also means women who have had abortions can't reach beyond their network to get support from others who have had abortions. (This contrasts with the one benefit of visible stigma, which is that groups such as racial minorities can build identity and community around shared social experience.)

Identifying groups of people as direct or indirect abortion beneficiaries doesn't mean every one of them is a closeted ally of pro-choice politics. Dr. Tate says that every day she provides abortions, at least one patient grabs her arm and says, "I just want you to know I'm not like those other women." Women who see their abortion as an *exception* to who they are, an aberrational event they want to distance themselves from rather than integrate, have another reason to not support abortion services or other people who will need them in the future. Not wanting to identify with other women who have abortions might also be a product of internalized stigma. Stigma separates "us" from "them." Rather than allowing new information to change a negative definition of "them" (e.g., "I'm a good person and I'm having an abortion, so maybe everyone else in the waiting room is like me"), these patients of Dr. Tate seem to be working overtime to stay on the "us" side.* Rape, incest, and me.

Some of Dr. Tate's patients come from a conservative neighboring state with restrictive laws and a lack of clinics that lead them to undertake over six hours of travel and a night in a hotel to have an abortion. Once during an election season, she told women from this state, "Remember this when you vote!" on their way out. "And they'd just look at me blankly—like, 'This won't be relevant to me then.' ... Many women I see feel they're exceptional, and they don't

* Some patients express abortion stigma in a different way—rather than distinguishing themselves from the other patients, they distinguish themselves from the clinicians. Researchers who interviewed 14 abortion providers from different facilities across a western state concluded that feeling "devalued" while serving a patient is a common challenge for people working in abortion clinics. As one provider put it, "I find it really stressful if patients are telling us how horrible we are. ... [W]hen you're working as hard as you can to give someone good service and they hate you, it's really hard." O'Donnell J, Weitz TA, Freedman LR. Resistance and vulnerability to stigmatization in abortion work. *Social Science and Medicine.* 2011;73:1357–1364, 1360.

care if abortion is legal for anyone else any other day. They think what got them in this predicament is unique."

Stigma helps to explain how a right that's so widely exercised can be so profoundly threatened. The number of American women who have an abortion every year is five times the number diagnosed with breast cancer every year, but you'll never see patients, family, and friends at "Fun Run for Abortion." The combined effect of the external stigma that keeps patients like Amelia silent, and the internalized stigma that makes some of Dr. Tate's patients cling to the idea they're completely different from every other abortion patient, is one reason the large number of Americans who are abortion patients or abortion beneficiaries haven't become a health advocacy group.

If people like Dr. Tate's pro-life picketer and Congressman DesJarlais don't want children, and if abortion is so stigmatized that no one wants to be an abortion patient, why don't more people prevent pregnancy with contraception?

Almost half of American pregnancies are unintended. Forty-five percent! (I live in a social circle of obsessive planners, so I found that number shocking too.) American women have 2.8 million unintended pregnancies a year, and 42% of them end in abortion. People on both sides of the abortion debate find common ground on the desirability of reducing unwanted pregnancies, 89% of Americans say they think contraception is morally acceptable, and contraceptive technologies are getting better. So why hasn't contraception eliminated our need for abortion?

Accidental pregnancy is the underlying condition patients in abortion clinics are asking doctors to remedy. One reason we have so many accidental pregnancies is the surprising number we have to prevent. "Natural fertility" is the number of babies a fertile woman would have if she were sexually active throughout her reproductive years and never used contraception. Demographers put this number at about 18 births.

The number of pregnancies a sexually active fertile woman needs to prevent depends on how many children she wants to have. In 1800, the average white woman in the United States had 7 babies.* In 2015, the average American woman had 1.8 babies. (Interestingly, this is close to the "replacement rate," the number that keeps population levels stable.) Assuming for a moment that the number of children American women currently have is similar to the number they want, that means two things: modern American women need to prevent more pregnancies than their predecessors, and that number is high.

Say Jane is a fertile woman who only wants two children. The average age of first intercourse for women in the United States is 17, so let's imagine that's when Jane begins having regular sex. (To avoid the distraction of sex stigma, let's say Jane's first partner, Leo, turns out to be the love of her life and quickly becomes her husband.) Jane and Leo don't just have to dodge the approximately 16 other pregnancies she's estimated to have without any contraception—they have to dodge more than that, because every month is a new opportunity to conceive. (Once you become pregnant, by definition you will only have one pregnancy in that nine-month period. If you're not pregnant, you have nine chances for an accidental pregnancy in the same time frame.) That's why demographers estimate that a fertile woman who relied solely on abortion for birth control would need up to 29 abortions to limit herself to delivering only two children.

Now let's be real: I'm going to guess most women don't have sex *every* month of their lives from age 17 to 45. But it's still helpful to understand that a fertile woman who wants to have only two children and no abortions, and has regular sex throughout her reproductive years, has to prevent somewhere between 16 and 29 pregnancies.

That's a tall order. Many try, but neither people nor contraceptives are perfect. Contraceptive failure rates come in two versions: perfect

* Black fertility rates weren't reliably documented until the 1850s.

use and typical use. "Typical use" accounts for average people's actual imperfect or inconsistent use of contraception over the course of a year. If 100 sexually active couples used no contraception for a year, researchers would expect 85 of them to get pregnant. If the same 100 couples used condoms perfectly, 2 would get pregnant. But with typical condom use, 18 of them will get pregnant. So condom use (both typical and perfect) dramatically reduces unintended pregnancy, but it certainly doesn't eliminate it. Perfect diaphragm use results in 6 pregnancies per 100 couples over a year; typical use results in 12. Perfect pill, patch, or ring use results in only 0.3 pregnancies in 100; typical use results in 9 pregnancies per 100 couples over a year.

Sometimes embarrassment about sex, or lack of power to insist on using contraception, keeps us from contraceptive perfection. Lack of access is a significant factor too. The most reliable methods of contraception, like the Pill or an intrauterine device (IUD), require a doctor's appointment. When financial, educational, or social barriers keep women from medical care, their only option is drugstore methods like condoms, spermicides, and sponges, which have higher failure rates. The reality of human imperfection, structural barriers to the most reliable methods, and occasional failure of contraception itself is underscored by the fact that 59% of women with unintended pregnancies report they used contraception the month they got pregnant.

Amelia had been using a NuvaRing, but a change in the source of her health insurance meant she had to go one month without it. Then, in the heat of passion, neither she nor Mike left her apartment to go buy a condom.

Amelia feels guilty about that. She was a 28-year-old with a college degree, and her mother was a health teacher who talked to her daughters about contraception, so she never thought of herself as someone who would get pregnant because she wasn't using contraception. Writer Leslie Jamison is another well-educated woman who didn't use contraception. In a book of essays, she describes the abortion she had while she was a graduate student at Yale with great detail, nuance, and emotional insight. Yet on this topic, she says only that she cannot "provide an adequate account" of why she "didn't use protection." Perhaps Leslie also surprised herself on this count; perhaps her own behavior doesn't make sense to her in retrospect either. But women like Amelia and Leslie have company: studies show that 41% of women with unintended pregnancies either did not use contraception, or did use contraceptives the year they got pregnant but had gaps in use of a month or longer when they were sexually active.

Here's the good news: contraception has gotten better. It's hard to know exactly how many abortions were performed before abortion was legalized, but it's estimated that there were approximately one million illegal abortions per year in the United States. Two years after *Roe*, in 1975, there were approximately one million legal abortions. The number of legal abortions peaked in 1990 at 1.6 million, then declined, until in 2014 there were 926,200. Putting these numbers in terms of lifetime incidence can make them more comprehensible. Abortion's prevalence in 1992 led researchers from the Guttmacher Institute to estimate that 43% of reproductive-age women in the United States would have one. In 2008, that estimate went down to 30%, and according to the latest data, in 2014 it went down to 24%.

Improvements in contraception play a large part in the recent drop. For example, the overall use of any method of contraception increased slightly between 2008 and 2012, but more important was the fact that the use of highly effective long-acting methods, particularly IUDs, increased from 4% to 12% between 2007 and 2012. When used consistently and correctly, contraception can be very effective. The two-thirds of American women who use it this way account for only 5% of unintended pregnancies.

Here's the bad news: contraception won't get us out of the abortion debate. We work to prevent lung cancer and heart disease by encouraging people to stop smoking and start exercising, and we can work to prevent accidental pregnancy by encouraging people to use contraception. But we won't accomplish perfect prevention in any area of medicine. Improvements in contraceptive education, access, and technology could reduce abortion rates even further, but contraception won't eliminate the abortion conversation completely.

So let's improve it. Our public abortion conversation feels thin. We've debated abortion for decades, yet the issue doesn't feel resolved or illuminated; it feels irreconcilable and repetitive. One reason the abortion debate feels unrewarding is it's grounded more in theory than practice. Our abortion debate largely excludes the people who actually live the policy and philosophy we've been debating. The number of American abortions is at an all-time low. And still, the current rate means 1 in 4 women will have an abortion.

So what might enrich the conversation? Prevalence is down. Now let's reduce paradox. Acknowledging ordinary abortion says nothing about whether it's a good thing or a bad thing; it says that discussing what's actually happening would be helpful.

Our public abortion conversation also suffers from a focus on law, and a confusion between law and ethics. Law is what you can and can't do, and ethics is what you should and shouldn't do. That doesn't mean there's no relationship between law and ethics. But being unclear about which conversation we're having makes it harder to discuss that relationship. In class I often draw this grid to clarify which analysis we're pursuing:

ABORTION

	Constitutional right?	Ethical action?
Yes		
No		

"Pro-choice" is a legal position that abortion is a right protected by the Constitution (as the *Roe* Court concluded), and/or a policy analysis that abortion should be legal even if it were left to the states. But saying you think abortion should be legal isn't the same as saying you think abortion is a good thing to do. Some pro-choice people think abortion is a morally neutral or morally good thing. Some are "abortion ambivalent"—strong defenders of the legal right who feel conflicted about the ethics of the choice.

And some people I know are pro-choice/anti-abortion: they agree with the constitutional analysis, or as a policy matter they think it's best for abortion to remain safe and legal, but they think abortion is immoral and would like to convince people not to do it.

The legal right to abortion is foundational. If it were up to me, the country's most prominent provider of contraception and abortion would be called Voluntary Parenthood. "Planned" is meant to signify "wanted," but not all unplanned pregnancies are unwanted. And "planning" is a value—a belief that it's better to lead with the head than the heart, a belief that life's best lived according to plans rather than fate or chance—that not everyone shares. "Voluntary Parenthood" identifies the true principle driving American pluralism—the belief that every citizen must be free to follow his or her conscience and chart the course of his or her own life.

Yet the legal reasoning that concludes individuals should be allowed to make pregnancy decisions privately is only step one. The second step in reasoning is the ethics conversation.

One type of ethics conversation focuses on individual cases. Ethical reasoning happens when the millions who privately choose abortion decide it is a moral act, or decide that it's "moral enough" to allow them to honor other imperatives. But abortion stigma means we usually don't get to hear their thought process, even if we're in the circle of people who love them. The silence of those who have chosen ordinary abortion is part of the reason abortion—as distinct from the value of "choice"—isn't defended as morally good to the same degree it is attacked as morally bad.

Another type of ethics conversation focuses on theories. You rarely hear someone say she or he is "pro-abortion," because that label is largely inaccurate. (Pro-choice advocates don't propose laws that would force women to abort wanted pregnancies, they don't erect fake prenatal care facilities to lure pregnant women into unwanted abortion counseling, and they don't picket actual prenatal care facilities urging women to think twice before they continue their pregnancy.) Yet the stigma of being labeled "pro-abortion" means people outside of philosophy departments rarely risk making the moral arguments in favor of abortion generally. For example, defenses of Planned Parenthood usually emphasize the fact abortion is a very small part of what it does, rather than arguing abortion is one of the many good things it does.

However, recent books offering affirmative moral cases for abortion suggest that's starting to change; for example, Katha Pollitt's *Pro: Reclaiming Abortion Rights* ("I want us to start thinking of abortion as a positive social good and saying this out loud."); Ann Furedi's *The Moral Case for Abortion* ("Whether a woman can be compelled to carry a fetus and give birth to a baby is just as much a moral question as those raised about the value of the fetus."); and Dr. Willie Parker's *Life's Work: A Moral Argument for Choice* ("I remain a follower of Jesus. And I believe that as an abortion provider I am doing God's work."). This is a trend we should embrace—because don't you want to hear the full range of arguments before you make up your mind?

How could we remedy the deficits of the American abortion conversation? Let's share more individual experiences, and let's talk about the full range of ethical theories. If we could talk to each other privately in a way that embraces the complexity of our lives and the nuance of our thinking, perhaps that enriched experience would lead to more reality and civility in our public abortion debates as well.

The rest of this book is intended to encourage and equip you to engage in respectful, productive, private conversation about your experience with, and opinion of, abortion. Sometimes we talk to learn. Sometimes we talk to persuade. And sometimes we talk simply to become known to each other, to confirm we live in the same moral universe, though we may never agree.

Chapter 2

Abortion Storytelling

Law, Masterplots, and Counter-Narratives

In a trial, lawyers function as competing authors. A story is a description of events, and lawyers construct different stories from the same facts hoping their narrative will prevail. Legal stories are required to be nonfiction, yet two factually true versions of the same event can be told differently enough that they lead to different conclusions.

Judges do their own version of this high-stakes storytelling: opinion writing is a type of advocacy intended to persuade colleagues and the public that their ruling and reasoning are correct. And in the opinions of the U.S. Supreme Court, the Justices writing the majority opinion and the dissent are often engaged in a narrative duel of their own.

The Supreme Court has considered various aspects of abortion law over the last forty-five years. However, three of those cases are key to understanding the constitutional right to abortion: *Roe v. Wade* (1973), *Planned Parenthood v. Casey* (1992), and *Gonzales v. Carhart* (2007).*

Roe, Casey, and *Carhart* are complex opinions that tell multiple stories, but I'm most struck by the story each tells about American

* The Court's most recent abortion case, *Whole Woman's Health v. Hellerstedt* (2016), is also important. It is discussed in Chapter 6.

abortion. In the Supreme Court's abortion story, the roles of protagonist (the main character, with whom we generally are meant to sympathize) and antagonist (the source of conflict or threat to the main character) change in each opinion. Thinking about perspective-taking in these Supreme Court opinions raises a good question for anyone interested in abortion storytelling: Whose story is it?

These Supreme Court opinions can also draw our attention to masterplots. That's what literary scholars call a culture's recurring stories. A masterplot is the bare bones of the story—for example, the details of "The Little Engine That Could" are very different from the details of Horatio Alger stories, but the skeletal plot of both is the same: hard work rewarded with success. Analyzing individual stories can be instructive, but new insights arise when stories are considered collectively. Which stories do we hear over and over again, and why do those particular stories have such staying power?

I begin by focusing on legal accounts of the American abortion story because these authoritative public tellings of it both reflect cultural masterplots and help create them. Reviewing these cases will also give readers unfamiliar with constitutional law some legal background.

Cultural masterplots can be instructive and useful. Masterplots play a powerful role in questions of identity, values, and our understanding of life. But a masterplot takes a story that's true for some and makes it the only story we can tell, the only story we're able to hear, the only story that counts.

Counter-narratives are stories that supplement or contradict a culture's masterplots, and when they're integrated into storytelling, they can weaken the power of prejudicial types. However, masterplots influence how we process new information. In an (often unconscious) effort to make the new story fit smoothly with the masterplot we already know, we sometimes supply connections that aren't actually in the new story, or ignore elements that are.

If internalizing cultural masterplots can blind us to counter-narratives, recognizing them for what they are and intentionally opening ourselves to counter-narratives can strengthen independent thinking. So after considering the Supreme Court's storytelling, I identify some abortion masterplots and consider counter-narratives that either amend them, or suggest alternative storylines.

The current abortion stories available to us are inadequate, and in some cases they're inaccurate. Stigma has suppressed many stories of ordinary abortion. Once they're told, collectively they have the power to create the more accurate, inclusive abortion masterplot we so desperately need.

ROE V. WADE (1973): ABORTION IS THE DOCTOR'S STORY

In *Roe v. Wade* the U.S. Supreme Court ruled that abortion is a constitutionally protected right. Before viability the Constitution prohibits state and federal legislatures from banning abortion, and after viability it prohibits them from banning abortion when pregnancy threatens a woman's life or health.

In the decision that established abortion as a constitutional right, plaintiff "Jane Roe" is introduced in about one sentence: we learn she's an unmarried pregnant woman in Texas who wants an abortion performed by a doctor, and she can't afford to travel to a state where that's legal. From there she functions as a placeholder for all women. The generic woman in *Roe*'s abortion story is threatened by unwanted pregnancy, and the opinion focuses on the negative aspects of delivering an unwanted child:

> Maternity, or additional offspring, may force upon the woman a distressful life and future. Psychological harm may be imminent.

> Mental and physical health may be taxed by child care. There is also the distress, for all concerned, associated with the unwanted child, and there is the problem of bringing a child into a family already unable, psychologically and otherwise, to care for it. In other cases, as in this one, the additional difficulties and continuing stigma of unwed motherhood may be involved.

But the woman isn't really the protagonist. Instead, Justice Harry Blackmun's majority opinion in *Roe* frames abortion as the doctor's story. In the *Roe* narrative, before viability "the abortion decision in all its aspects is inherently, and primarily, a medical decision, and basic responsibility for it must rest with the physician." The physician is the hero, the main actor who makes decisions and rescues the pregnant damsel in distress. The *Roe* Court says its decision "vindicates the right of the physician to administer medical treatment . . . ". None of the maternity issues the Court listed in the section quoted above is strictly medical. Yet "[a]ll these are factors the woman and her responsible physician necessarily will consider in consultation."

The *Roe* Court ruled that fetuses don't fit within the Constitution's use of the word "person," and the opinion doesn't paint the fetus as a character or personify it as an active agent. Instead, *Roe*'s abortion story frames pregnancy and parenthood as antagonistic states or events, natural forces that can threaten a woman like a storm and its aftermath. The fetus itself is framed as an unknowable entity that's outside the jurisdiction of the courts and, before viability, beyond the authority of the legislature.

Dissent: The *Roe* decision was 7–2, and Justice Byron White's short dissent (joined by Justice William Rehnquist) tells a different abortion story: the story of the callous, cavalier woman. He does this by using the word "convenience" four times in a two-and-a-half-page opinion. He says:

- The *Roe* majority is deciding the Constitution "values the **convenience**, whim, or caprice of the putative mother more than the life or potential life of the fetus . . . ."
- "The Court apparently values the **convenience** of the pregnant mother more than the continued existence and development of the life or potential life that she carries."
- The Texas statute in question "denies abortions to those who seek to serve only their **convenience**, rather than to protect their life or health."
- Reasons women might want to end pregnancies include "**convenience**, family planning, economics, dislike of children, the embarrassment of illegitimacy, etc."

This dissent concludes that the claim in *Roe* is that "any woman is entitled to an abortion at her request" "for any one of such reasons [listed above], or for no reason at all . . . ."

PLANNED PARENTHOOD V. CASEY (1992): ABORTION IS THE WOMAN'S STORY

Almost 20 years later, the Supreme Court considered a case asking it to overturn *Roe v. Wade,* and the Court refused to do so. Instead, it affirmed *Roe*'s ruling that the Constitution prohibits states from banning abortion before viability. Yet Justice Sandra Day O'Connor's majority opinion in *Planned Parenthood v. Casey* tells a very different abortion story from that of *Roe.**

* The proper term for what Justice O'Connor wrote in *Casey* is "plurality opinion"—reasoning that wasn't endorsed by over half the judges on a panel, but received the most votes among those on the side of the winning outcome. I refer to it here as a "majority opinon" for simplicity because, with the exception of the undue burden standard, the sections of the opinion I'm analyzing were supported by five Justices.

The plaintiffs in *Casey* are five abortion clinics and a group of doctors, yet the generic woman is the protagonist of *Casey*'s abortion story. She's a person who has "urgent claims . . . to retain the ultimate control over her destiny and her body." As Justice John Paul Stevens put it in his concurrence (a separate opinion joining and supporting the majority opinion): "The authority to make such traumatic and yet empowering decisions is an element of basic human dignity. . . . [A] woman's decision to terminate her pregnancy is nothing less than a matter of conscience."

In the abortion story told by the decision that affirmed abortion as a constitutional right, a woman granted a right to abortion is an empowered person who gets to choose her role in society: "The ability of women to participate equally in the economic and social life of the Nation has been facilitated by their ability to control their reproductive lives." *Casey* expands the story to include women as a group, and it includes men by using the word "people": "[F]or two decades of economic and social developments, people have organized intimate relationships and made choices that define their views of themselves and their places in society, in reliance on the availability of abortion in the event that contraception should fail."

The pregnant woman denied an abortion is still a sad victim of circumstance in *Casey*, but instead of focusing on the burdens of parenting an unwanted child as *Roe* did, *Casey* emphasizes the burdens of pregnancy and giving birth. A woman who carries a pregnancy to term is "subject to anxieties, to physical constraints, and to pain only she must bear. . . . Her suffering is too intimate and personal for the State to insist, without more, upon its own vision of the woman's role, however dominant that vision has been in the course of our history and our culture."

The antagonist in the *Casey* abortion story is a State that would use its power to force women into social roles that differ from what individual women want for themselves. Justice Blackmun states this vividly in his concurrence: "By restricting the right to terminate pregnancies, the State conscripts women's bodies into its service. . . ."

The *Casey* opinion doesn't frame the protagonist of the abortion story as a patient. Instead she's "a woman" or "the woman," and the physician is largely absent. Unlike *Roe*'s abortion story, in which doctors rescue women in distress, in *Casey*'s abortion story the Supreme Court depicts itself as a bodyguard that stands between a restrictive State and "[a]n entire generation [that] has come of age free to assume *Roe*'s concept of liberty in defining the capacity of women to act in society, and to make reproductive decisions. . . ."

The shift from *Roe*'s focus on the physician to *Casey*'s focus on the woman receiving medical care in the context of her whole life is consistent with other changes in American law, medicine, and culture in the nineteen years that passed between the two decisions. The patients' rights movement and the rise of medical ethics in the 1970s and 1980s were fights over who gets to define "the good," and patients won—meaning they, not doctors, ultimately get to decide what's best for their bodies in the context of their own lives and individual values. For example, when *Roe* was decided, patients didn't have a legal right to refuse lifesaving medical interventions such as ventilators. By the time *Casey* was decided, this kind of patient right was clearly established.

The fetus is a very minor character in *Casey*'s abortion story. Consistent with *Roe*'s ruling that fetuses aren't persons within the reach of courts or legislatures, in *Casey* fetuses are brought to capital-L"life" only through the beliefs of people who have not chosen to have an abortion: "[Abortion] is an act fraught with consequences for others: . . . for the spouse, family, and society [some of whom deem abortion] nothing short of an act of violence against innocent human life; and, depending on one's beliefs, for the life or potential life that is aborted."

However, the same opinion that portrays a woman who controls her reproductive life as a fully realized citizen who can participate equally in economic and social life also includes a second part that allowed significant restrictions on her abortion rights. For the first nineteen years after *Roe*, virtually no restrictions were allowed before viability. Then *Casey* adopted the "undue burden" rule—a new standard of review that allowed the recent flood of state restrictions on pre-viability abortion. In Chapter 6, I discuss the politics and impact of these regulations collectively. But in the realm of storytelling, the *Casey* opinion highlights the difficulty of multiple authors producing a single narrative voice: in order to affirm the core holding of *Roe*, liberal Justices Stevens and Blackmun had to live with the undue burden standard advanced by moderate Justices O'Connor, Anthony Kennedy, and David Souter.

Dissent: The *Casey* decision was 5–4, and the four Justices in the minority wanted to overturn *Roe*. (Justices Rehnquist and White, who held that position as dissenters in *Roe* nineteen years earlier, were now joined by Justices Antonin Scalia and Clarence Thomas, who were not on the Court when *Roe* was decided.) Justices Rehnquist and Scalia both wrote dissents primarily responding to the majority's arguments on the constitutional issues, and its story of the contested role of the Court and *Roe* in politics. But each also makes a small contribution to writing the American abortion story. Justice Rehnquist disputes the majority's assertion that reproductive control is central to women's economic and political lives: "Surely it is dubious to suggest women have reached their 'places in society' in reliance upon *Roe*, rather than as a result of their determination to obtain higher education and compete with men in the job market, and of society's increasing recognition of their ability to fill positions that were previously thought to be reserved only for men." And Justice Scalia shares his impression that abortion's legalization has eliminated abortion stigma: "*Roe* created a vast new class of abortion consumers and abortion proponents by eliminating the moral opprobrium that had attached to the act. ('If the Constitution *guarantees* abortion, how can it be bad?'—not an accurate line of thought, but a natural one.)"

GONZALES V. CARHART (2007): ABORTION IS THE FETUS'S STORY

Gonzales v. Carhart came thirty-four years after *Roe* and fifteen years after *Casey*. The case was not a direct challenge to the right to abortion, but it was significant because it was the first time the Court upheld a ban on a particular procedure for performing an abortion, and because the ban did not contain the life-and-health exception that had previously been required of all restrictions.

In *Carhart,* the Court reviewed a federal law prohibiting a procedure doctors call intact dilation and extraction (intact D&E) and others call "partial birth" abortion. This law doesn't stop anyone from getting an abortion. Instead, it makes it illegal to use a method the professional organization of obstetricians and gynecologists (ACOG) said was safer for patients in some situations. It allows the procedure when a woman's life is in danger, but does not include an exception for her health. In *Carhart,* the Court ruled that the federal "Partial-Birth Abortion Ban Act" did not violate the constitutional right to abortion itself. The majority opinion was written by Justice Kennedy.

The fetus is the main character in *Carhart*'s abortion story. (The terms "unborn child," "infant life," and "a child assuming the human form" are also used, but the term "fetus" predominates.) In this narrative the fetus is a victim in distress—it's threatened by untrustworthy doctors, and rescued by Congress. The *Carhart* opinion quotes a nurse who "witnessed" an intact D&E. A nurse present in a professional capacity would usually be said to have "assisted" or "participated in" a procedure; the verb "witnessed" frames the physician like a defendant in a criminal case.

A fetus cannot narrate its own story. Who has the authority to speak for any particular fetus, or for fetuses generally? In the majority opinion, the nurse reports "the baby's arms jerked out, like a startle reaction, like a flinch, like a baby does when he thinks he is going to fall." Here the fetus is a baby who comes alive narratively as a character with a point of view assigned to it by the narration of the nurse—it has expectations about the future (it's startled) and thoughts (he thinks he's going to fall).

In the *Carhart* abortion story, Congress rescues the fetus and protects the integrity of the medical profession. Women can still choose second-trimester abortions, but their doctors can't choose between procedures to accomplish that goal: "The law need not give abortion doctors unfettered choice in the course of their medical practice . . . ."

The doctor is back to being a central figure in the abortion story, but in 2007 it's as the antagonist to the fetus. *Carhart* moves the character of the doctor away from *Roe*'s fatherly Marcus Welby figure and toward a villainous Dr. Mengele figure. These doctors aren't identified by their medical specialty (obstetrician-gynecologists, family physicians, or surgeons) but as "abortion doctors," a label the minority opinion calls pejorative. The word "convenience" returns too, except now applied to doctors instead of patients: the medical judgments of these physicians are dismissed as "preferences" motivated by "mere convenience." In bioethics, if a choice between procedures is not seen as an issue of medical judgment about patient safety, it must be an issue of patient autonomy. But in the *Carhart* abortion story, "abortion doctors" can't be trusted to share facts their patients might want to know: "In a decision so fraught with emotional consequence some doctors may prefer not to disclose precise details of the means that will be used, confining themselves to the required statement of risks the procedure entails." Therefore, the Court permitted Congress to eliminate the option of using this procedure entirely.

Women are also victims in *Carhart*'s abortion story—not of unwanted parenting (*Roe*) or unwanted pregnancy (*Casey*), but of abortion itself: "Whether to have an abortion requires a difficult and painful moral decision. … While we find no reliable data to measure the phenomenon, it seems unexceptionable to conclude some women come to regret their choice to abort the infant life they once created and sustained. … Severe depression and loss of esteem can follow." Women might also become victims of unscrupulous doctors who take advantage of their naïveté: "It is self-evident that a mother who comes to regret her choice to abort must struggle with grief more anguished and sorrow more profound when she learns, only after the event, what she once did not know: that she allowed a doctor to pierce the skull and vacuum the fast-developing brain of her unborn child, a child assuming the human form."

Dissent: The *Carhart* decision was 5–4. Justice Ruth Bader Ginsburg's minority opinion (joined by Stevens, Souter, and Stephen Breyer) reasserts *Casey*'s placement of the woman as the main character in the American abortion story. It contends that cases challenging abortion restrictions "do not seek to vindicate some generalized notion of privacy; rather, they center on a woman's autonomy to determine her life's course, and thus to enjoy equal citizenship stature." (Of course this contest over the proper protagonist in the abortion story, the woman or the fetus, mirrors one framing of the American political debate.) The dissent argues that the majority's portrayal of women is an outdated story: characterizing women as needing special protection, and accomplishing this by depriving them of the right to make autonomous choices, "reflects ancient notions of women's place in the family and under the Constitution—ideas that have long since been discredited."

MASTERPLOTS AND COUNTER-NARRATIVES

These three Supreme Court opinions strengthened or helped to create several abortion masterplots; here I consider three of those. Stories that contradict these masterplots—counter-narratives—might inspire us to amend or reject them.

Masterplot 1: Abortion is always a difficult decision

One cultural masterplot is that deciding whether or not to terminate a pregnancy is always a difficult decision. In 1992, Justice Stevens referred to abortion as a "traumatic decision" in his concurring opinion in *Casey*. In 2007, Justice Kennedy asserted it on behalf of the *Carhart* majority—"Whether to have an abortion requires a difficult and painful moral decision"—and Justice Ginsburg repeated it in that case's woman-centered dissent: "The Court is surely correct that, for most women, abortion is a painfully difficult decision. But. . . ." (Then she cites the compelling evidence that abortion does not hurt mental health.)

The "difficult decision" masterplot serves those who oppose abortion (and perhaps those who are conflicted about it) by suggesting everyone exercising the right must at least pay a penalty of emotional distress. It also serves those who support the right, by suggesting the women who exercise it are considering opponents' arguments, an expression of respect that might help appease them. Less obvious is how the "difficult decision" masterplot hides a moral assessment of embryos and fetuses.

Why, exactly, might an abortion decision be difficult? A pregnant woman who assigns embryos high moral value would likely find weighing that against her own interests difficult, and deciding that it must be sacrificed painful. But a pregnant woman who does not share this belief about embryos would be unlikely to struggle in this way. Stories of ordinary abortion illuminate how the "difficult decision" masterplot answers the moral question the abortion right supposedly leaves to women.

At a bioethics conference I attended, a panelist repeated this masterplot, stating that abortion was always a difficult decision. In the question-and-answer period, philosophy professor Bonnie Steinbock went to the microphone and offered a counter-narrative. She responded not with philosophical theory, but with her own story of becoming accidentally pregnant at age 26. It's extremely rare for academics to spontaneously assert the insight of intimate experience in front of hundreds of colleagues, and it was an arresting moment for me as an observer. As she later wrote:

> Frankly, I am sick and tired of this particular piety. The decision to have an abortion is not inevitably agonizing, wrenching, or traumatic—at least, not in my experience. … At the time, I was living with a man with whom I was very much in love, but who I knew was not as much in love with me. I did not think about the embryo at all; for me, a five-week-old embryo is not the kind of being to which one can have moral obligations. Rather, I thought that if I had the child, my real purpose would be to get my boyfriend to marry me, and that would be incredibly manipulative. Thus, for me, the abortion decision was not difficult. I do not wish to minimize the anguish an abortion decision causes many women. Indeed, there are situations in which I would find abortion terribly difficult, despite my pro-choice leanings. If we'd been engaged or married, but not ready to have a child, I would have had a lot more trouble deciding what to do. Nevertheless, to assume that the decision to have an abortion is always difficult not only ignores the experiences of women like me, but worse, implies that women who do not find the decision difficult are somehow deficient psychologically or morally. And that is a canard women can live without.

Amelia (mentioned in Chapter 1) also didn't find her abortion decision difficult. She's an actor, not a philosophy professor, so she puts it more plainly: "I think it was me looking at my life and being like, What do you want your life to look like? And can it still look like that with a child right now? And it would not. And I decided I did not want that. And I was okay with that." Earlier I said one reason I think of the majority of abortions as "ordinary" is because they bring a woman's body back to its baseline state. Amelia captures the existential aspect of that idea—abortion returned her *life* to its baseline state.

Amelia's counter-narrative both reveals and challenges a variation on, or subplot of, the "difficult decision" masterplot: a story that says abortion is always a life-altering event. Amelia's story suggests that is not always true.

Amelia confirmed the drugstore pregnancy test with her doctor (she was between six and eight weeks along, she recalls) and went to the clinic he recommended. It was only two miles from her apartment, and there were no protesters. She had a good experience there: "All of the doctors and people I came in contact with were extremely supportive and not judgmental in any way, so that it made it very easy to be like, you're right, this is a mature and intelligent decision and these people are going to take care of me." The man she created the pregnancy with arrived bearing milkshakes, he drove her home, and she took the night off from the play she was appearing in. The next night she was back at work.

"I feel like it should have been a monumental decision," she told me. "In my head it was like, 'This is going to be the thing. This will be huge, right?' You're taking a life—it felt like it was supposed to be monumental." But that wasn't how it actually felt to her. "I wasn't terribly sad about the experience, because I knew it was the right thing to do for me. It was like twelve hours of my life went by in a weird way, and then everything went back to normal. It wasn't more than that."

Why didn't Bonnie and Amelia find their abortion decisions "difficult" or "painful"? Because, as Bonnie says explicitly and Amelia implies, they do not think an embryo has a moral status that requires them to keep it alive. Stories of ordinary abortion don't just teach us abortion is common. They also open the door to the moral reasoning behind each one.

Okay, fine. Amelia wasn't torn up about her abortion. But that could change, right? She might regret it later.

"Abortion regret" is another variation on, or subplot of, the "difficult decision" masterplot. Abortion is *such* a difficult decision that even if you feel confident it's the right one, you might change your mind later. As noted above, in *Carhart* Justice Kennedy wrote: "[I]t seems unexceptionable to conclude some women come to regret their choice to abort the infant life they once created and sustained." Driving through my home state of Indiana, I've seen this masterplot repeated on a billboard—enormous letters proclaiming, "Many women regret their abortion."

The possibility of regret doesn't distinguish abortion from the rest of medicine. Without perfect knowledge of the future, the possibility a well-informed patient might later wish he or she had not chosen back surgery, a kidney transplant, or a panoply of other procedures can never be eliminated. The prevalence of ordinary abortion underscores this point—when millions of people choose a medical procedure, it stands to reason that they won't all have the same reaction to it later.

However, recent data suggests the regret narrative isn't representative. A research project known as the Turnaway Study followed 667 women having abortions at 30 facilities across the country, interviewing them every six months to see what they thought and felt about their experience over time. "Women in this study overwhelmingly felt that the decision was the right one for them: at all time points over three years, 95% of participants reported abortion was the right decision, with the typical participant having a >99% chance of reporting the abortion decision was right for her."

A decision that's "right" isn't always easy. The Turnaway researchers also asked this group how much difficulty they had in deciding to seek an abortion, and their responses covered the spectrum: 13% said their abortion decision was very easy, 18% somewhat easy, 15% neither easy nor difficult, 27% somewhat difficult, and 27% very difficult.

Earlier I said one reason an abortion decision might be difficult is if the woman assigns a high moral value to embryos. A second reason is difficult social circumstances. I think of negative emotions about circumstances as "situational regret." A patient who chooses knee replacement instead of joint pain might regret choices he made years before on the football field; a patient consenting to painful cancer treatment might regret she ever started smoking. Similarly, some abortion patients might regret getting pregnant, or might be sad or angry* about the circumstances that make having a baby the wrong choice for them at this time. If these patients could travel back in time to change the behaviors that created their medical needs they would; but they see the medical intervention as the better of two undesirable options.

"Decisional regret" is what worries us—a patient's feeling that knowing how things turned out, if she could travel back in time she would make a different medical decision. The Turnaway Study suggests this is uncommon in abortion, but sociologist Katrina Kimport offers a story that illustrates it. She interviewed 18 abortion patients who reported "emotional difficulty" around their abortion. Seventeen

* These are normal emotions, not mental health problems. The Turnaway Study also measured mental health indicators every six months for five years after an abortion, and found no evidence abortion harms women's mental health. Biggs MA, Upadhyay UD, McCulloch CE, Foster DG. Women's mental health and well-being 5 years after receiving or being denied an abortion. *JAMA Psychiatry*. 2017;74(2):169–178.

of these women had situational regret (what Kimport calls "head vs heart" conflicts) and one had decisional regret.

Brandy was 20 years old when she became pregnant. She sat down with her mother and went over the positives and negatives before she chose to terminate. A year later she said, "If I could go back and change it, I wouldn't have had the abortion. … No matter if the father was there or not, no matter if I was going to be a single mom struggling, I would've not had the abortion. … I think I would be much more happier now."

It's hard to know what Brandy could have done differently—it sounds like she thought things through carefully with someone she trusted. Yet looking back, she now wishes she'd made a different decision. My heart goes out to Brandy and every woman like her. What should we make of decisional regret, what should we do? A concept from a different area of bioethics, disability ethics, could help.

"The dignity of risk" is a concept articulated in the 1970s to challenge clinicians' impulse to withhold options from people with disabilities unless good outcomes were guaranteed, and it's shorthand for the fact there is no opportunity for success without a right to failure. All our medical decisions are really best guesses—"I think this will be best for me, but only time will tell." (We know this is true of other important life decisions, like marriage or job choice, too.) Instead of infantilizing patients, disability ethics argues that granting them the dignity of risk means that informed decisions they later regret are viewed as an opportunity to learn, grow, and develop resilience. The dignity of risk reminds us that competent adults must be allowed to take chances and risk pain in pursuit of a better life. Decisional regret isn't a clinical complication, it's a feature of life.

Is it worse to regret an abortion decision than other decisions? (Or if decisional regret is possible either way, as it logically must be, is it worse to regret a decision to abort, or to carry a pregnancy to term?) The debate these questions inspire reveals the degree to which concerns about abortion regret might ultimately circle back to an estimation of the moral value of embryos and fetuses (which I explore in Chapters 4 and 5).

If abortion decisions aren't always difficult or painful, why don't we hear more stories from women on the other side of this spectrum, women like the 31% in the Turnaway Study who said the decision was "very" or "somewhat" easy? Amelia and I talked on a deck overlooking the ocean as the sun set. I told her I thought thousands of women might have stories like hers they were keeping to themselves. She set down her wineglass and volunteered a deeper reason we rarely share feelings and experiences that contradict the "abortion is always a difficult decision" masterplot:

> I think the reason you don't hear it is because it feels so casual and cavalier, and as smart, educated, somewhat financially stable women, who wants to admit that? Admit that I made a mistake about life and I chose to get rid of it. Nobody wants to admit that. But the sad fact is sometimes it's just not right. And I don't think it's bad, but a lot of people think it is. And it feels like a weird—I don't know if "privilege" is the right word, or "entitlement," but it's like, "Oh, you just get to get rid of your mistake, you just get to take care of that?" And I think that's an embarrassing way to look at it. I think it's still a stigma that it feels casual. . . . But it was me, so I know there's feelings involved, and there's life involved, so it wasn't robotic.

I don't think Amelia's decision was casual. I think it was confident.

Decisions aren't difficult when circumstances match what you've already thought through. Bonnie says she "did not think about the embryo at all" during her abortion decisionmaking process, but the next half of the sentence ("for me, a five-week-old embryo is not the kind of being to which one can have moral obligations") reveals that she'd already thought about embryos a lot—enough to have reached a considered value judgment about her moral obligations (or lack thereof) before her accidental pregnancy.

Similarly, people know that sex can sometimes lead to pregnancy, so having sex might prompt some to think through their feelings about abortion. If accidental pregnancy does occur, their response might seem obvious: of course they're going to have the baby, or of course they're going to have an abortion. If their current feelings or circumstances conflict with the values they've already clarified, the decision might be difficult.

The "abortion is always a difficult decision" masterplot underscores the moral seriousness people making this decision are expected to have. But people who don't struggle with an abortion decision are not necessarily less morally serious than those who do—they're just less undecided. Someone who is clear about who she is, what she values, and what she wants is not casual. She is confident.

Yet there are few examples of this type of counter-narrative. Bringing a child into the world is of great moral consequence, yet we don't frame the decision to *have* a child as a difficult decision people always struggle with. So why wouldn't some abortion decisions feel similarly obvious? We recognize the archetype of the confident, responsible, morally thoughtful woman who quickly knows motherhood is right for her and has no regrets, but when you substitute the word "abortion" for "motherhood," that woman is unrecognizable. Amelia earlier said she'd made "a mature and intelligent decision." Yet masterplots that depict abortion as an inevitably difficult, life-altering decision ripe with the possibility of regret may have contributed to her complex feelings.

Listening to Amelia talk, I said it sounded like she felt guilty that she doesn't feel guilty about her abortion. "Yeah. That's fair! I don't feel bad about it, I think it was absolutely the right decision for me to make. So there's absolutely no guilt about it. If anything, I feel guilty about the way I started that relationship." Amelia became teary. "It was embarrassing for me to know I had had that experience with someone who maybe I liked him more than he liked me."

Essayist Leslie Jamison (also mentioned in Chapter 1) describes a version of these complex feelings after her abortion during graduate school: "I felt guilt that I didn't feel more about the abortion. . . . I felt the weight of expectation on every moment—the sense that the end of this pregnancy was something I *should* feel sad about." Later she writes that she did experience some sadness, and explores the possibility that she "was attaching long-standing feelings of need and insecurity to the particular event of this abortion." She describes crying about what she calls her "voluntary loss" on an unexpected occasion: "I felt simultaneously like I didn't feel enough and like I was making a big deal out of nothing."

Dr. Willie Parker identifies a related masterplot—"Abortion is always a tragedy"—and in *Life's Work: A Moral Argument for Choice,* he offers his experience as an abortion provider as a counter-narrative. In doing so, he describes a large number of women whom I'd call confident.

> One of the cultural falsehoods that I most rail against is this: each and every abortion is a terrible tragedy and every woman who chooses to have an abortion is therefore a tragic figure. In this popular narrative, women are helpless victims—and not clear-eyed individuals making a sensible choice to benefit themselves and the people around them. I know, from seeing women every day, how far this is from being true. Most of the women I see are utterly matter-of-fact about what they're doing. They're on my table because they need to be. . . . It may be difficult in a misogynist culture to regard women who freely choose sex and who freely choose to have abortions when needed as free agents taking their lives into their own hands. But the alternative is to

see them as less than fully human and requiring of paternalistic intervention.

Women like Bonnie, Amelia, and Leslie may be exactly who Justice White had in mind when he wrote about "convenience abortions." These women are adults. They're educated. Their partners were perfectly nice men. And yet—still—they don't want to have a baby.

Justice White said that the claim in *Roe* was that "any woman is entitled to an abortion at her request" "for any one of such reasons [listed above], or for no reason at all . . .".

What does it look like for someone to have an abortion "for no reason at all"? Both life and storytelling tell us it's impossible to do even the most boring action for *no* reason. Sit down, stand up, drop off the dry cleaning—there's always *some* reason. "No reason" is brutally trivializing. "No reason" is the analysis of a narrator who can't reach someone's interior life. It means: no reason I can see, no reason I can understand. Or it means: I *do* see what's motivating this character, but her reason isn't one I value, so I will use my power as narrator of this story to reduce it to zero—no reason at all.

Here's the reason: Bonnie, Amelia, and Leslie had abortions because having a child at that time or in that situation didn't fit their vision of their future, and they do not believe embryos have a moral value that outweighs that.

The majority and minority opinions in *Roe v. Wade* juxtapose the "serious abortion," a medical decision between a woman and her doctor, and the "convenience abortion," a personal decision a woman makes for herself. I can't say whether *Roe* created this contrast or just captured a sensibility that already existed, but our public abortion conversation seems to have maintained it. Amelia hasn't read Justice White's forty-five-year-old dissent, she doesn't agree with his framing, and she didn't use the word "convenient." But when Amelia said other people might consider her action "casual and cavalier," this echo of the *Roe* dissent suggests she has internalized a cultural masterplot that instructs her to feel bad and keep quiet.

Masterplot 2: Abortion is a women's issue

The masterplot that portrays abortion as a "women's issue" is pervasive. The majority opinion in *Casey* is centered on this premise, and it is repeated in cultural examples too numerous to count.

Legally, the "women's issue" masterplot is accurate. Socially, it's incomplete. Biologically, pregnancy can't happen without a man's participation. And the majority of unwanted pregnancies occur in relationships: 88% of women who have abortions in the United States are dating or married to the man they got pregnant with.

So where are men in the American abortion conversation? The way in which all these boyfriends and husbands* are largely absent from abortion discourse—both literally as speakers and imaginatively when we picture American abortion—is another way in which our public abortion conversation doesn't match the reality of lived experience. We've allowed a legal discourse that properly focuses on individual rights to substitute for a social and political discourse that reflects reality. Thinking about ordinary abortion could help us correct that.

In Chapter 1 I introduced the concept of "abortion beneficiaries"—people who didn't terminate a pregnancy themselves but benefited from the fact someone else did. The first time I shared my idea of men as abortion beneficiaries in an academic presentation,

* In the context of medicine and public health, the word "partner" is a wonderfully nonjudgmental word for anyone a patient has had sex with. Outside that context, it's cold. In common discourse, "partner" can subtly suggest sex is just a string of one-night stands. Words like "boyfriend" and "husband" aren't what every heterosexual woman chooses, but in this context they remind us that for many women seeking abortion, pregnancy occurs within romantic relationships.

a professor named Paul stuck around afterward. "This is just personal," he said as he scanned the room to confirm it had cleared. Then he told me his college abortion story. Paul is in his late 50s with a bushy red beard and sparkly demeanor. He was shy, thoughtful, and sweet as he spoke. "I guess I should talk more about how I benefited from that."

Some would say men like Paul are largely absent from public discussion about abortion because abortion decisions aren't up to them. Legally that's true—a man can't force a woman to have an abortion when she wants a child, and he can't force her to have a child when she wants an abortion. And in *Casey*, the Supreme Court ruled that states can't require women to notify their husbands about an abortion.

Yet women usually do tell their male partner about their abortion: 82% of abortion patients surveyed in waiting rooms report the man they got pregnant with knows about their abortion. Within this group of patients, 79% report he was supportive of it, 12% said he was "neither supportive nor unsupportive" or that they weren't sure, and 9% said he was unsupportive. (The survey didn't define "unsupportive," so it is unclear to me if these women were saying their partners opposed the abortion, or that their partners were unhelpful.) This suggests what one might guess about functional couples—many men either participate in abortion decisionmaking, or are on the same page with a girlfriend, wife, or sexual partner who made a unilateral decision.

Twelve percent of abortion patients said they were *not* in a relationship with the man they got pregnant with. (The majority of this group, 61%, still report this man knows about their abortion, and a majority of that group, 64%, report that he was supportive.) The professor I spoke with after my presentation is a member of this group—a man who was not in a romantic relationship, but knew about his partner's abortion and agreed with her decision. Two years after Paul told me his story I was still thinking about it. Why hadn't personal experience motivated this liberal, educated man to speak up? Fully expecting him to decline, I wrote an awkwardly apologetic email asking if there was any chance he'd be willing to share more, and for quotation. He surprised me by responding immediately: "It would be a pleasure."

Paul went to an elite college in the late 1970s, and in his senior year he and five friends shared a house. He was particularly good friends with Jan, and one night after he'd gone to bed this roommate surprised him by joining him. The evening was "an outlier, it wasn't a meaningful encounter," and Paul doesn't remember things being different between them afterward. Later, Jan told him she was pregnant, and that she was going to have an abortion. "It was a matter-of-fact, 'I am, and this is what's going to happen'" kind of conversation. What did he think or feel when she told him? "I was like, 'Of course that's what you're going to do, what else would you do?' It wasn't something I wrung my hands about."

After college, life unfolded pretty much as Paul hoped. He got a Ph.D. and landed a terrific job. He fell in love and married a wonderful woman at age 36. He and his wife quickly had two kids, whom it's clear he adores as he describes the ways they're now flourishing in college. He hardly thought about his abortion experience until decades after college. A friend Paul made later in life also had a youthful one-night stand that resulted in pregnancy, but his friend's partner chose to continue her pregnancy. Paul's friend has participated in his child's life over the years, but it's always been a difficult situation. "And it's been fascinating to appreciate the obvious, which is that, um, my life could have been so radically different if Jan hadn't done what she did. I'm so grateful—my life went so much better because I got lucky and did not have to either take responsibility for raising a child, or live with the guilt of not taking responsibility for sharing in the raising [of] a child. It's just shocking."

It's inevitable that some couples will disagree on reproductive decisions. Some men will be upset at becoming a father, and some will be upset at not becoming one. The voices of men who feel wronged by their partner's abortion decision are occasionally part of the discourse. (For example, I've seen pictures of men protesting abortion carrying signs saying "I Regret My Lost Fatherhood.") That makes it even more important for us to hear from the majority of boyfriends, husbands, and partners of women who have an abortion—the thousands of men each year who feel comfortable, relieved, or pleased with the abortion decision their partner made, with or without his participation.

Abortion is an individual legal right—the Constitution frees women from state control, which is often a proxy for male control. But socially, abortion is not only sometimes a shared experience, it's often a shared benefit. A more nuanced political conversation would account for the difference between the legality of abortion—which is, and must remain, a woman's individual right—and the social experience of abortion, which is often more of a "couples' issue" than a "women's issue."

But first we need examples. Before telling me his story, Paul had mentioned the event only to two male friends and his wife. "Three times in 36 years. That's kind of"—he sighed—"that's not many times." Why not? "I haven't had the courage to talk about it because it's a painful memory—it's a shameful memory. Not the fact I got someone pregnant, or the fact of the abortion. But . . ." Paul sputtered. "I didn't offer to go with her to get it. . . . I just—at the time, my head was so far up my ass, I really didn't—can you imagine—it just—none of it really registered. It never—I didn't know that it would be a big deal for her to go and actually get this procedure that it was obvious that she wanted to get. . . . But I should've understood that the procedure was a big deal and that I should've been present for it. And that I didn't has really haunted me."*

Talking to Paul wasn't that different from my conversations with women who are personally comfortable with their abortion decisions but don't mention them to many others. Paul is staunchly pro-choice, and his wife writes checks to groups like Planned Parenthood and NARAL. He told me that after he and I first chatted after my presentation,

> it did occur to me that I should try to write an op-ed and come out, and I decided against it. I just—I don't want to go there. But I think it would be a good thing if some man did. Because it is weird. We get at least 50% of the benefit, and it's a horrible mistake to forget that or ignore that or to not recognize it. … [P]eople like me do have some sort of obligation to do more than write checks. It is a remarkable gift to have this ability to make a decision to postpone parenthood or avoid it altogether so I should be doing more. Contrary to the course of this conversation, I'm actually a rather private person and I—I am not really eager to make this an issue I talk a lot about publicly, because more than anything I think my children are at an age where that's not exactly what they need.

I don't think anyone has an obligation to reveal his or her personal life for a political cause. Yet I wonder: what would happen politically if a large proportion of all the men who feel like Paul thought abortion was their issue too? I have a feeling the right to abortion might suddenly seem a lot more secure.

* I wondered if Paul was projecting the "difficult and painful" masterplot on his friend's abortion. No—he said this because years later Jan said something that led him to believe it actually was difficult for her.

In Chapter 1 I identified another group of abortion beneficiaries: all the men and women who never had an accidental pregnancy, but have been able to enjoy sex as part of their romances and marriages because they weren't constantly afraid of contraceptive failure. Framing abortion exclusively as a woman's issue also lets millions of men in this group of beneficiaries off the hook.

Elise Belusa is a lovely woman in her early thirties who manages academic research projects in a liberal city. She invited me to a campus coffee shop to discuss her international abortion research. In the course of conversation she made an offhand comment that she'd seen an increase in sexism in recent years, but she wasn't sure what had changed: the world, or her ability to spot sexism. When I asked for an example, Elise said she'd been on several dates with men who learned she worked in abortion and responded, "It's a woman's body and that's completely her decision." I was taken aback. How is that an example of sexism?? Elise said she knows that's their way of showing support—"It's what they've been trained to say"—but it irritated her for reasons she wasn't quite able to articulate. We explored it further, and finally uncovered what bothered her about the "It's completely your decision" response. It's lonely.

The comments Elise's dates made are another example of legal discourse displacing interpersonal discourse. "Your body/your choice" is a liberating legal framing that asserts a woman's individual right to control her body. But when the legal framing of abortion as a women's issue is repeated in a social context between people who could conceivably make love someday, it sounds more like a message of abandonment than support. Socially, "your body/your choice" contributes to inequality by shifting all the burden of the possible consequences of sex to the woman. Think how different it might sound to Elise if these young men took moral responsibility for abortion by responding to her job with something like, "Yes, abortion can be the right thing to do." Shared moral responsibility means you won't have to carry that Scarlet A alone. It also suggests shared social responsibility, in which a partner volunteers to walk alongside her in whatever emotional, practical, and financial ways she wants.*

I asked Elise if she thought the young men who said, "I support whatever you choose" really meant that they would support her if she had an accidental pregnancy and chose to have a child. She laughed. "Absolutely not. They're assuming you'd have an abortion. So that's why it feels like a transfer of responsibility." As Paul did in his youth, these men get to avoid both unwanted fatherhood *and* the social stain of abortion. And by repeating abortion's legal framing in a social setting, they manage to sound progressive as they do it. That is not to say the law is wrong—I think the law is correct. It's to say allowing the legal conversation to dominate or replace all other types of abortion conversation is a mistake.

A progressive view of gender roles expects modern men to share responsibility in areas like birth control and parenting. Applied to abortion, this view might suggest that people who start an unwanted pregnancy together end it together. For many, that will mean going through the event together. For all, it could mean sharing moral responsibility for the act, social responsibility for destigmatizing the choice, and political responsibility for keeping abortion available. The same principle applies to men who have not experienced an unwanted pregnancy but are able to have sexual relationships without fearing they must necessarily result in fatherhood. Amending the "women's issue" masterplot could help men understand how they benefit from abortion's legality, and why those who believe they benefit should work to keep it that way.

Feminist support of abortion rights pushes our cultural gaze outward, from a fetus in isolation to a woman and fetus in relationship.

* An obligation to offer is not the same as an entitlement to do—of course some women will prefer support from people other than the man with whom they became pregnant.

Perhaps it's time to look even further, from a pregnant woman in isolation to a pregnant woman and her male partner in relationship, when that is the case. This has nothing to do with law—men have no legal claim to any more information or decisionmaking power than their female partners decide they have earned. But stories of ordinary abortion might help us understand abortion as something that's often (though certainly not always) a "couples" issue. Then a next generation of advocacy could continue to reject men's control without surrendering a moral claim to men's practical and political contributions.

Masterplot 3: Abortion is about sex

Gigantic pictures of bloody fetuses hang from a bus parked on the main square of a Southern college campus. It's "The Genocide Awareness Project" making its yearly visit. Several people in their 50s, 60s, and 70s stand in front of the bus yelling that abortion is murder and will send you to hell. They urge anti-abortion flyers on students on their way to class, and when a young woman walks by without acknowledging them, one of the men yells after her: "Slut!"

Why would "pro-choice" mean "promiscuous"? When a graduate student in my seminar described this moment from her college days, her classmates didn't think a lack of interest in anti-abortion flyers said anything about a young woman's sex life. But they were familiar with the idea that it did.

The cultural masterplot that abortion is about sex is used to diminish the significance of the right. Abortion is framed as something that allows "sex without consequences," or something that "cleans up" after irresponsible sex.

Yet sex commonly occurs in the context of dating and marriage. So why isn't abortion understood as an issue of romance, relationships, and family?

As noted above, the vast majority of women having an abortion (88%) report they are in a relationship. Half of this group are living with a man (15% are married and 29% are cohabiting), and the other half (44%) are in a dating relationship. Sixty-two percent of abortion patients have been with their boyfriend or husband over a year, and 26% have been with him for under a year.

Numbers aren't counter-narratives, and statistics aren't as sticky as stories. But when the masterplot doesn't match the research, it's important to remember that statistics are stories reduced to data points. These numbers help us understand abortion as a predictable consequence of dating and marriage. That doesn't make it ethical—that's a separate part of the conversation. It makes it unsurprising.

Learning that the majority of abortion patients are in romantic relationships made essayist Leslie Jamison's use of the pronoun "we" and the way she marks time through love (versus meeting or dating) stand out to me: "We'd been in love about two months when I got pregnant. I saw the cross on the stick and called Dave and we wandered college quads in the bitter cold and talked about what we were going to do. ... I remember wanting Dave to be inside the choice with me but also... I needed him to understand he would never live this choice like I was going to live it." Later, Jamison describes their experience going to Planned Parenthood together to end her five-and-a-half-week pregnancy, and sharing a bed the following nights as she recovered.

These statistics also attuned me to another counter-narrative I'd never considered: abortion as a family issue. Are mothers the abortion clinic clientele you imagined? Me neither, until I read the research.

The majority of abortion patients in the United States are already mothers (59%). A third of women who have abortions have two or more children (33%) and a quarter of them have one child (26%).

Martha Ashe was a 30-year-old mother in Georgia when she remarried, and she and her new husband had four children between the two of them. "This was in the early days of blended families—it was hard for kids of divorced parents. My ex and his ex each lived in town, and the kids were splitting their time between households, and the school couldn't figure out how to do the directory with kids having different last names and different parents." Six weeks after the wedding she discovered she was pregnant. "We wanted to have a child together, to celebrate being together. But six weeks? It seemed like just a catastrophe for putting this family together." Martha is a soft-spoken professor who's in her seventies now. She leaned back and looked at the ceiling as she recalled the past. "We were all still getting used to this new thing. I remember staring out the kitchen window at the trees thinking we *could* do this, but what about the children? This would throw a monkey wrench in the whole thing."

Martha's husband, who was also a professor, felt the same way. Their decision to terminate their accidental pregnancy felt obvious and simple. They did it and had no second thoughts. "Then after we'd all been together for a year and it had been successful, we made up our minds to have a baby in the summer," when their college was on break and they could both be home for three months. It was the early 1970s* and Martha's accidental pregnancy had occurred while she

* Although Martha Ashe had her abortion in 1971, it was a legal abortion. Before *Roe v. Wade* was decided in 1973, approximately one-third of states had liberalized their abortion laws to varying degrees, and 1.3 million legal abortions were reported to the Centers for Disease Control and Prevention (CDC) between 1970 and 1972. In 1970 four states generally allowed abortion on request before viability, but New York was the only one of the four states that didn't have a residency requirement. As a result, in 1972 over 100,000 women left their home states to terminate a pregnancy in New York. Martha was one of these women. Abortion was illegal in Georgia, so she flew to a New York physician recommended by her Georgia physician for a safe, legal, but quite expensive, abortion. Gold RB. Lessons from before Roe: Will past be prologue? *Guttmacher Report on Public Policy*. Mar. 2003;6(1).

was using an early version of the modern IUD (a "Lippes Loop"), so now she was using birth control pills. She planned to go off them in the fall. But that summer Martha had her second unintended pregnancy. "Let me near sperm and I'll conceive," she laughed. "My doctor couldn't see anything wrong—I had switched to the Pill, but an allergy medicine might have made it less effective?" So their daughter Clare was born in March instead of June, and Martha got a tubal ligation to ensure she wouldn't have anymore "pregnancy adventures."

Earlier I used the term "moral intuition." Moral intuition is an emotional or subjective indication of appropriate or ethical behavior in a given situation. Whether it is a valid source of judgment is a topic of debate. Ethics professor Sabine Roeser's theory of moral intuition posits that our emotional attitudes can form a practical way to understand the validity of ethical beliefs. She rejects the idea that moral reasoning is an either/or proposition, objective or emotional, saying that we need intuitions and emotions in order to have objective moral knowledge. She proposes a cognitive theory of emotions in which emotions are a prerequisite for a rational practical decision, rather than mere "gut reactions" that can't form the basis of moral reasoning.

As Dr. Parker noted, some paint women as "victims" of abortion who don't understand what they're doing.* This framing insults all women, but it's particularly insulting to the 59% who are already mothers. Previous pregnancies have given the majority of abortion patients an experiential understanding of embryonic potential and fetal development. Their evaluation of—or, at minimum, intuition about—the moral status of embryos and fetuses is implicit in their choice.

* This stance refuses to grant what we might call "the dignity of disagreement." Disagreeing with the reasoning or conclusion of women who choose abortion respects them as thinking people. Instead, this Orwellian move categorically reframes disagreement as misunderstanding. It's an offensive attempt to maintain the speaker's supremacy by foreclosing even the possibility of dissent.

Martha Ashe wasn't a woman who couldn't feed another child, she was a woman with true choice. Perhaps you think women like Martha—economically comfortable married women who actually want another child—shouldn't end an accidental pregnancy because of its timing, and that is positively your prerogative. What this story tells you is that Martha and her husband assessed the moral status of embryos differently from you. They assigned more weight to the emotional interests of their existing children than to the interests of their embryo. If they had thought the moral status of their embryo was very high, they would have dealt with the downsides of bringing the first one they created to maturation.

Sex creates pregnancy, so of course abortion is "about" sex in some ways. But framing abortion as *exclusively* about sex demeans the role sex often plays in people's lives. This realization about the role of sex is part of what led to one of the rare instances in which the Supreme Court reversed itself. In 1986, in *Bowers v. Hardwick*, the Court held a state's decision to make gay sex a criminal offense was not prohibited by the Constitution. The case that reversed that ruling, *Lawrence v. Texas* (2003), begins by quoting the earlier opinion:

> [The *Bowers* Court said] "The issue presented is whether the Federal Constitution confers a fundamental right upon homosexuals to engage in sodomy" ... That statement, we now conclude, discloses the Court's own failure to appreciate the extent of the liberty at stake. To say that the issue in *Bowers* was simply the right to engage in certain sexual conduct demeans the claim the individual put forward, just as it would demean a married couple were it to be said marriage is simply about the right to have sexual intercourse. ... When sexuality finds overt expression in intimate conduct with another person, the conduct can be but one element in a personal bond that is more enduring.

The masterplot that depicts abortion as just about sex similarly demeans the claims of women seeking them. Later in the *Lawrence* opinion, Justice Kennedy quotes *Casey*, the case that affirmed *Roe* in 1992:

> [Opposition to homosexuality] has been shaped by religious beliefs, conceptions of right and acceptable behavior, and respect for the traditional family. For many persons these are not trivial concerns but profound and deep convictions accepted as ethical and moral principles to which they aspire and which thus determine the course of their lives. These considerations do not answer the question before us, however. The issue is whether the majority may use the power of the State to enforce these views on the whole society through operation of the criminal law. "Our obligation is to define the liberty of all, not to mandate our own moral code." *Planned Parenthood of Southeastern Pa. v. Casey.*

COMING OUT WITH COUNTER-NARRATIVES

Why don't we hear more stories of abortion as a straightforward decision, as a couples issue, as a family issue? Abortion stigma is a strong inhibitor, but it would be a mistake to blame it for everything. Identity and the mechanics of storytelling are two other factors.

After we talked about his college roommate's abortion, Paul said he wondered if he should "come out." His use of that concept is resonant, and it's tempting to draw an analogy between the abortion rights movement and the gay rights movement. If everyone who ever had an abortion or who benefited from its availability "came out" to family, friends, and colleagues, surely the stigma around abortion would decline.

However, people connected to an abortion experience and LGBTQ people differ in important ways. Abortion is an event, not an identity. Think of it in terms of TV shows: a gay character can live through multiple seasons, but "woman (or couple) who has an abortion" isn't a character, it's a plot line. Converting an event into an identity is reattaching that Scarlet A—to say when we look at you, your abortion is all or most of what we see.

The difference between identity and event has narrative significance. Coming out as lesbian or gay can be done through An Announcement. It can also be done more subtly by intentionally integrating identifying language into daily conversation. Imagine this office exchange:

BOB : I finally saw that movie everyone's talking about.
LISA : Yes! Sue and I saw it on our first date.

Bob has options—he can talk about the movie while he processes (or shrugs at) new information about his colleague's sexual orientation, or he can choose to follow that conversational thread to learn more. Lisa has options too—natural opportunities for smoothly inserting identifying language occur frequently, which means Lisa can choose a moment she feels safe, or has the energy and time for the potential follow-up, to do it.

Weaving an event like abortion into casual conversation is harder:

BOB: Sorry I'm late, my wife has terrible morning sickness.
LISA: Oh, I know what that's like. I mean, I don't have kids—I had an abortion.

You're feeling sorry for Bob, aren't you? Lisa too! They both might be frozen in conversational amber. It's a hard statement to ignore, it's hard to engage with, and because it happened in the past it's hard to know its relevance to today. My examples are silly, but ask yourself: is there any smooth way for Lisa to share the fact she's had an abortion? My point is simply that even if the political benefits of coming out with abortion stories are comparable to coming out with sexual orientation, and even if one is willing to take the plunge, the storytelling obstacles to each are distinct.

Finally, the collective power of coming out as a lesbian or gay man could benefit you personally in the long run, as well as others in that community. But if you think you will never have or be involved in another abortion, coming out about your abortion means risking social stigma so others can benefit from abortion's legality, accessibility, and acceptability in the future. And because not having a child maintains one's life as it was, people with positive or neutral abortion experiences might not view it as a momentous occasion they feel moved to bring up.

The storytelling analysis is different for abortion providers. Abortion isn't a single event for them, it's part of their professional identity. It's challenging work, so it might be fair to guess no one does it unless they find it meaningful and resonant with their personal identity as well. The simple fact that abortion providers spend a significant amount of their time doing this work might also create more natural opportunities for storytelling.

Yet providers don't discuss it much either. The prevalence paradox, which focuses on women who have abortions, was discussed in Chapter 1. Physician Lisa Harris and colleagues offer a neat parallel called "the legitimacy paradox," which describes the cycle of stigma and silence abortion providers face. Public discourse stigmatizes abortion providers as dangerous, deviant, or illegitimate. Abortion stigma and the constant threat of violence and personal harassment lead providers to discuss their work only within small circles. Their silence means abortion work is not seen as the type of work a neighbor, soccer club acquaintance, or colleague would do. So despite the fact a highly trained, compassionate cadre of health care professionals have for forty-five years provided safe abortion care that many millions of American women desperately wanted, providers continue to be stereotyped as rogue doctors whom the state is justified in regulating out of existence.

Kara Evans is a nurse who kept her job to herself. She's spent many years partnered with a doctor to provide abortions in a Southern state with laws that lead the Guttmacher Institute to classify it as "extremely hostile to abortion." Her neighbors knew her primarily as a mother, and that's how she wanted it.

Then Kara was involuntarily "outed" by Operation Save America (the new name of Operation Rescue). They distributed flyers to everyone in her neighborhood. This happened in 2012, but she still has one of the flyers. They feature a photo of her smiling face and her name next to a picture of a fetus exposed by fetal surgery. The headlines say "ADOPT AN ABORTION WORKER," and that Kara "is complicit in the murder of hundreds of precious children every year." Below the picture it gives her office and home address. Operation Save America cruised her neighborhood in a billboard truck with images of a dismembered fetus on the side, visited her neighbors door-to-door, and picketed her house once. Their website claimed they mailed 800 flyers.

Kara was horrified. This was exactly the exposure she always feared.

Then days passed. Weeks. And her feeling about the flyer changed to amazement.

"I didn't get a single negative reaction," she exclaimed. About five neighbors commented. "It was either 'thank you for what you do,' or 'I don't agree with what you do, but no one messes with my neighbor.' Some of them even offered to call the police and file a complaint." The flyer encouraged its recipients to write her at her home address to ask her to stop working for the clinic. No letters? "I got one very nice letter thanking me for my work and encouraging me to continue to be a provider." And that was it.

Kara and the doctor she works with almost always have picketing at their office, and they did see an increase in protesters in the weeks after the flyer. The doctor was subjected to a similar attack. He lives in a smaller town, and Kara reports he got a mixed reaction. Most of his neighbors were supportive, but he also got some cold stares and avoidance. His high-school-age children got comments in school from some classmates, and even from some teachers.

Four months later, Kara had to visit everyone in her neighborhood for another reason, and she was anxious. After all, no comments didn't mean she wouldn't see a new chilliness from neighbors who used to be friendly. "I braced myself for the comments or dirty looks," she said. Then she went door-to-door with her daughter to sell Girl Scout cookies.

How'd it go? "Not even one."

Five years have passed, and being "out" hasn't disrupted Kara's work or life any further. Every situation will be different, and no one should ever be "outed" involuntarily. But Kara's experience helps us remember that our fear of negative repercussion isn't the same as the fact of negative repercussion. Stigma's power lies in the way it makes fear as controlling as fact.

Is there a *Will & Grace* of abortion? It would have to be a show about abortion providers, because the medical procedure that's an event for patients is a professional identity for the people who do it every day. Given all providers already do, it's too much to ask for them to also "come out" if they would prefer not to. But humanizing them and their patients through fictional characters with recognizable lives would accomplish similar goals, and focusing on provider characters might be the only way to sustain patient plot lines without converting an event into an identity.

Women are entitled to be the authors of their own life stories. Autonomy is having the authority to say, "I don't want a major plot twist or an additional character right now." I care about what stories women get to live, as well as what stories they get to tell. The right to end an unintended pregnancy—regardless of whether you choose to exercise it, regardless of how you feel about it afterward, regardless of whether you keep it to yourself or shout it from the rooftop—is an essential part of that.

Ordinary abortion is a large part of abortion experience and a small part of abortion narratives. But I think there's much to be learned from the ordinary story we overlook. Today many people experience abortion as a safe medical procedure that returns their bodies and lives to baseline. In Chapter 4 I review a spectrum of approaches to abortion ethics. The story of ordinary abortion reminds us that abortion *experience* also occurs on a spectrum, from utterly wrenching to fairly painless to welcome relief, with many falling in between.

Make no mistake, some contemporary abortion stories are far from ordinary. Too many women are shamed, delayed, and made to pay more for the procedure by laws designed to impose these burdens (which I discuss in Chapter 6). Too many women must fear violence and brave picket lines that make what *could* have been a routine medical procedure a traumatizing event. And some are completely denied access to abortion because they can't afford to pay for a medical procedure that's often not covered by private insurance or public aid. Other people have easy access to abortion, but struggle with sadness about the life circumstances that led to an unwanted pregnancy or that made them feel unable to care for a child they really wanted. All these stories matter.

However, stories of ordinary abortion help us bring the numbers I discussed in Chapter 1 out of the shadows, reminding us that in the

United States, many people want or need an abortion, and many people have one. The prevalence paradox implies no one is talking about abortion, but of course that's not the case. People who *have* abortions aren't talking about it much. That creates a storytelling vacuum, which others fill. When the masterplot doesn't match the data, we should consider the possibility that it's abortion opinion masquerading as abortion experience.

So which is it? Are abortion decisions difficult or easy? Are they life-altering or not? Is abortion a women's issue, or a couples issue, or a family issue? Is it about sex or isn't it? It's all of those things. Yet a masterplot takes a story that's true for some and makes it the only story we can tell.

Until new stories of lived experience replace it.

Chapter 3

Abortion Conversation

Mapping a Minefield

A seventeen-year-old girl in a small town in Utah didn't want to be pregnant, but she was—she was seven months pregnant. So she paid a guy she met at the 7-Eleven to beat her up, which she hoped would induce a miscarriage. Twenty-one-year-old Aaron Harrison took her $150, then took her to the basement of his parents' house and kicked her in the belly.

Aaron Harrison pleaded guilty to attempted murder, but at sentencing a judge ruled murder—killing "another human being"—wasn't the right crime. Instead, the judge thought a different statute better fit the facts of the case, one that prohibited the attempted killing of an "unborn child." The prosecutor argued Harrison should get the murder statute's longer penalty because of this line in Harrison's written confession: "She started to ask me if I knew anyone to kill the kid for her and I said, 'No I don't.' " So, the prosecutor argued, Harrison's own word choice showed he believed what was in her belly was a "kid," which falls under Utah's murder statute.

Who was right? Was she carrying "another human being"? A "kid"? An "unborn child"? Something else?

This shocking case is truly extraordinary—it's an attempt at self-abortion, *and* it occurred after viability. I consider it here because this neon case illuminates vocabulary questions raised by those that are less visible.

Words have serious consequences in law, but that's true in everyday conversation too, especially when the topic's abortion. Americans have a lot of different words for what pregnant women carry in their bellies. You'd think broad vocabulary would facilitate meaningful discussion, but on this topic it seems the first obstacle to it.

The abortion debate is about more than control of conception. It's also about control of conceptualization. Abortion politics shapes our language on the topic in ways both obvious and insidious, and choosing between contested words has become a minefield for the well-intentioned. As a result, even sincere people pursuing respectful discussion of abortion have a hard time capturing moral sensibilities, medical realities, and lived experiences in the same words. And feeling like "you can't say anything right" leads sane people with lots to contribute to leave the conversation in frustration, or to dodge it completely to avoid pointless sparks.

We can't communicate without shared language. If you want to talk about abortion, think of this chapter as a map to help you make it across this linguistic minefield intact. Which words are most (and least) conducive to productive discussion about abortion?

Life: For some the key word in the abortion conversation is "life." That's the word used in *Roe v. Wade*: "We need not resolve the difficult question of when life begins. … [T]he judiciary, at this point in the development of man's knowledge, is not in a position to speculate as to the answer." Scientifically speaking it was odd to say the judiciary can't speculate on this, because in 1973 biologists knew the same thing they know today: "life" exists at conception. Sperm, eggs, and zygotes (combined sperm and egg in its first days) are all made of living cells. Some add the modifier "human," but that only marks membership in the species *Homo sapiens*. So saying a woman is pregnant with "human life" only clarifies she isn't carrying a lizard.

But limiting the language of life to scientific definitions makes it deceptively simple. Philosophically, the word "human" isn't just a reference to our species' DNA. In everyday conversation "human" is often synonymous with "person," which casts the term "human life" in different light. The same is true for the word "life": in *Roe* it couldn't have meant only biological life, because after the Court said it didn't need to "resolve the difficult question of when life begins," it went on to say, "When those trained in the respective disciplines of medicine, philosophy, and theology are unable to arrive at any consensus . . . ." If the court is looking to philosophy and theology for answers, it too must mean "life" in its larger sense. So one reason words like "life" and "human" can be confusing is they have different meanings in different fields like biology and philosophy.

Potential life: This term could be understood as an attempt to reconcile biology and philosophy in one term. "Potential life" is confusing to scientifically minded people: adding "potential" seems inaccurate or repetitive, since a zygote, embryo, or fetus already is life. But the modifier "potential" can be read as marking a shift from "life" as biological fact (small-l life) to "life" as moral concept (capital-L life). Understood this way, "potential life" is biologic life that *could* become a member of the moral life in the future, but hasn't yet done so. Which is logical as an idea, and confusing as a term.

Person: This term is contentious because it also has a double meaning. "Person" is like "life" in this sense, but instead of philosophy versus science, "person" pits philosophy against law. The Constitution protects "persons," and *Roe v. Wade* is very clear that fetuses are not constitutional "persons" at any point in pregnancy:

> The Constitution does not define "person" in so many words. . . . [*Roe* then lists 16 uses of the word person in the Constitution.]

> None [of these uses] indicates, with any assurance, that it has any possible pre-natal application. All this, together with our observation, *supra,* that throughout the major portion of the 19th century prevailing legal abortion practices were far freer than they are today, persuades us that the word "person," as used in the Fourteenth Amendment, does not include the unborn.

So according to the Supreme Court, constitutional personhood only begins at birth. Of course a fetus could have moral status without legal standing, but when philosophers and theologians talk about whether fetuses are "persons," lawyers become anxious that word will drift into constitutional conversation without further analysis. You could try to clarify that you're using the word only in its philosophical sense, but calling an embryo or fetus a "person" also doesn't feel quite right socially: no one argues this additional "person" qualifies pregnant women for the carpool lane or a tax deduction.

Human being: The prosecutor in the Utah case called what Harrison kicked a human being (which is what the Utah murder statute prohibits you from killing) because Harrison referred to it as a "kid." Yes: kids (children) are human beings, and any fetus in a woman's belly is human. But does that make a fetus a human *being*? A corpse is human, but I wouldn't call it a human being. A clump of liver cells might be human, but they're not a human being. "Human" seems static and biological, a question of DNA. "Human being" seems active and socially defined. The term "human being" doesn't appear in the Constitution, so it doesn't have the legal meaning of "person." But in ordinary conversation "human being" is synonymous with "person," and that gives the term a social significance that sounds the same legal alarms noted above. "Human being" seems synonymous with "one of us," which is one of the questions abortion discussions seek to answer: "When is a fetus one of us?" Or, "At what point is it enough like us that it shouldn't be destroyed?" And starting with a term that carries its own conclusion is not conducive to conversation.

Kid: Aaron Harrison called what he kicked a "kid," and even this word isn't as simple as it sounds. Doctors would say he was wrong—medically, as long as it's floating inside a woman's body it's defined as a fetus. So why haven't I ever been invited to a "fetus shower"? Because at some point people who plan to carry a pregnancy to term start using the word that anticipates the social status coming around the bend, and that word is "baby." Some cultures with high rates of infant mortality don't name babies for months after they're born—infants aren't made full family members until it appears they'll survive. Perhaps America's low infant mortality rate leads us to apply the same logic in the opposite direction. In wanted pregnancies, socially many people make a fetus a full member of their family after the point in pregnancy when it seems they'll survive. But it's a mistake to conflate social roles within families and legal status within society—my mom still (accurately) refers to me as her child, but that social role in my family shouldn't make me ineligible to vote.

Potential child: This term is a variation on both "kid" and "person"—a "potential" kid or person. "Potential child" is scientifically and socially accurate (if this pregnancy continues it will result in a child), but it's provocative because it's a stealth carrier for a legal argument: "You can't kill a child, and this is a potential child, therefore . . ." But if it's right to identify and grant rights based on biologic potential, then children should be called "potential adults" and given driver's licenses, and adults should be called "potential corpses" and given funerals.

Unborn child: The judge called it an "unborn child." This term is illogical when used before an embryo or fetus can survive outside the womb (before approximately 6 months), because much more than just delivery stands between it and being a child—if it was born, it would die. But the fetus in the Utah case was viable so at one level "unborn child" was accurate: if the Utah teenager had gone into natural premature labor, what she delivered would be called a child.

However, what women deliver is more commonly called a baby, so perhaps "unborn baby" is the more accurate version of this concept. Does "unborn baby" make an embryo or fetus sound smaller, more dependent, or more morally ambiguous, than "unborn child"? If we're looking forward from that baby's development, why stop at child? "Unborn adult" is as accurate as "unborn child," but that doesn't suggest someone needing our care and protection.

"Unborn child" (or "unborn baby" or "unborn adult") also asserts an answer to a contested question: the moral significance of location. Does exiting another's body, having that umbilical cord cut, and surviving independently mark a morally significant status change? To some, the claim that an entity that lives inside another person's body is just a baby that hasn't yet been born completely erases the woman and the hard work her body is doing to nourish it.

The pregnancy: One term not raised by the Utah case is one obstetricians often use: "the pregnancy" or "her pregnancy." This refers to everything in the uterus—the embryo or fetus, plus the yolk sac or placenta, umbilical cord, and amniotic sac—because an embryo or fetus can't survive without these other elements. So "the pregnancy looks healthy" means every element is working, and abortion is called "pregnancy termination" because it removes everything in the uterus. This term acknowledges that before viability, "the fetus" cannot survive without "the pregnancy." Saying Harrison "ended her pregnancy" sounds different because "her" explicitly expands the focus past the fetus to include the woman in which it lives, and "pregnancy" connotes a process, or a state a woman occupies.

Below I list the terms I've mentioned so far for naming what pregnant women carry.

Fetus, embryo, or zygote (depending on age)
Life
Human life
Potential life
Person
Human being
Kid/child
Baby
Potential child
Unborn child/unborn baby/unborn adult
The pregnancy (or her pregnancy)

I've heard several people say, "Eskimos have, like, seventeen words for snow." The number varies, but all who say it nod sagely at the idea that you know something's important to a culture when they have lots of different words for it. None of our words for the … intrauterine traveler? … say whether abortion is ethical or should be legal. But every one of them seems to be the first step toward different conclusions, so of course they're contested. These linguistic gymnastics are part of what makes it hard even to start a conversation about abortion.

But years of teaching medical students about this topic has required me to start the conversation, and I've tried to make careful choices. I avoid starting with words that contain conflicting scientific, legal, and moral concepts, such as "life," "human," and "person," because that makes it easy for people speaking in good faith to be misunderstood. These multiple meanings also create ample opportunities for intentional sleight of hand. (For example, veering from scientific meanings to moral meanings in the same sentence: "Fetuses are human, human beings have moral status, therefore fetuses have moral status.")

To me, medical terms describing current stages of development seem like accurate starting points for conversation—words like "embryo" or "fetus"; "viable" or "nonviable." As a general term, "prenatal life" seems pretty neutral as well. Scientific terminology is not "pro-choice" except when it is similarly abused as a trump card (such as declaring "It's a fetus!" and stopping there, as if using the medical word exempts the speaker from arguing what moral status should flow from that fact). Other terms can be introduced into the conversation later, after the freight each carries has been identified and agreed on by the discussants.

"Fetus" is often used as shorthand for what pregnant women carry throughout pregnancy. Medically speaking, this is inaccurate. For ten weeks after a woman's last period, it is called an "embryo." Some believe an embryo has a different moral status from a fetus; some do not. To include people who think those entities are imaginatively or morally different in important ways, I use the medically accurate term when we're talking about abortion at a specific point in pregnancy, or the combined term "embryos and fetuses" when referring to the entire pre-viability period when abortion is legal. The fact that 80% of abortions occur within ten weeks of a woman's last period (eight weeks after conception) is why I sometimes refer to the "debate about the moral status of embryos."

Finally, I try to skip the "the." "The fetus" is an idea—a cultural abstraction and a political football. I prefer grammar that acknowledges bodies, because it signals a discussion that at least attempts to be grounded in experience or medicine rather than politics. We don't typically discuss "the woman"; we discuss women generally, or a woman specifically. I find it a more helpful parallel to discuss fetuses generally, or a fetus specifically, and to reserve "the fetus" for when I actually mean to refer to it as a cultural icon.

People with a religious worldview might say starting with medical or scientific words like "embryo" or "fetus" is far from neutral because these words already separate body and soul, stripping human creation of its mystery and grandeur. But I don't claim neutrality, I claim plurality: in our pluralistic society, bodies are a shared assumption in a way that ensoulment isn't, and if we don't start with a shared language, we can't talk at all. Feminists might say starting with these words is misleading, because they already separate women from that which they nourish, framing embryos and fetuses as independent entities rather than dependent entities subsumed in a term like "pregnant woman." But I don't claim completion either: focus on a piece doesn't preclude mindfulness of the whole, and for some people, or some discussions, focusing on embryos or fetuses is necessary.

How we think shapes how we talk, and how we talk shapes how we think. That's why terminology is contested ground in the abortion conversation. But all of our under- and over-inclusive words for embryos and fetuses make me wonder: Is it really that helpful to have seventeen words for snow? Or is the point rather that when you talk about something complex and important you need a range of words to describe it, each of which captures an important element, because none of them can encompass it all?

In the Utah case, serious criminal consequences revolved around this poignant linguistic dance. Aaron Harrison was first sentenced to the lesser term (five years) for attempted killing of an "unborn child" because the judge wasn't persuaded by the prosecutor's argument in favor of killing "another human being." The prosecutor appealed, and the Utah Supreme Court held Harrison's original charge and plea to the crime of attempted murder was correct, because he attempted to kill an unborn child in a manner other than a medical procedure. So the lower court reinstated the plea bargain, and Harrison was sentenced to 1–15 years for second-degree felony attempted murder.

The seventeen-year-old girl (identified in court documents only as J.M.S. because she was a minor) pleaded no contest* to solicitation

* A no contest (*nolo contendere*) plea has the same effect as a guilty plea—conviction and sentencing—but it's different because the defendant doesn't admit fault. Formally speaking, with this plea they neither admit nor dispute the charge.

to commit murder and was sentenced to juvenile corrections until she was twenty-one. Four months later the judge reversed himself: her new lawyer successfully argued that she hadn't broken any laws, because in Utah a woman can't be held criminally liable for seeking an abortion for herself. So legally, the judge determined the word relevant to her action was "abortion," not "murder," and she was released. The prosecutor appealed this decision as well, and the Utah Supreme Court ruled that a solicited assault was not an "abortion" because it is not a "procedure," and it gave the prosecutor discretion to press criminal charges against her.

The basement assault did not terminate J.M.S.'s pregnancy. She later delivered a healthy baby, which was removed from her custody and adopted by relatives.

Incensed that J.M.S. went free, the Utah legislature quickly responded with a bill defining self-abortion at any point in pregnancy as homicide. The revised version of this bill signed into law by the governor amended Utah's definition of criminal homicide to include women who cause the death of their "unborn child" by a reckless or criminally negligent act that is intentional or knowing. This law makes intentional miscarriage of "an unborn child" homicide "at any stage of its development"—even before viability, when abortion with a doctor would be legal.

There's no question that a pregnant woman being kicked in a basement is horrific for everyone involved. But the legislature's response to this unusual case means every Utah woman who has a miscarriage is at risk of the word "patient" becoming synonymous with the word "suspect."

A term that could be used to describe Utah's legislative response to this case is "moral panic." A moral panic happens when an individual or episode that deviates from the norm is defined as a threat to social order, a threat to "life as we know it." It's only one incident, but when a moral panic is triggered that one event invokes a wider radius of fear, disgust, and strong responses than single cases usually do. There's an intimate relationship between media and moral panics: media are necessary for spreading news of outrage and fear, and sometimes the media generate these feelings in search of ratings. Other times, politicians fill this role, generating these feelings in search of votes. Politicians, media figures, and others who benefit from this panic are sometimes called "moral entrepreneurs." The case of J.M.S. is rare—you almost never hear about women trying to hurt themselves to end an advanced pregnancy. But in Utah, perhaps it suddenly felt like pregnant women might be secretly clobbering their swollen bellies all over the state, and only a law like this can (and must! and will!) stop that.

When a case this outrageous and sad occurs, it's only natural to want to do something. But what's the best response? If the goal is to prevent similar situations in the future, I'd begin by trying to understand why it happened this time. What could make a teenager so desperate that she'd risk her own life to end a pregnancy by hiring a stranger to kick her?

J.M.S. was poor. Not "can't buy new shoes" poor; she lived in a rural house without running water or electricity. She was facing abandonment. She told police she solicited the assault after her boyfriend threatened to leave her if she didn't get an abortion. (News reports didn't say much about the role J.M.S.'s parents did or did not play in her life.) This "boyfriend" was a convicted felon who later faced charges of using minor J.M.S. and another teen in child pornography.

None of this is an excuse for what J.M.S. did. What she did was wrong, and she shouldn't have done it. But there's a difference between reasons and excuses. Excuses make a person forgivable. Reasons make them comprehensible.

J.M.S.'s fetus was vulnerable because J.M.S. was vulnerable. It appears as if she had a difficult life and limited choices long before she became pregnant. So although her case includes pregnancy, it's "about" more than that. J.M.S was a minor in need who does not seem to have gotten significant resources and support from her community or her country until she tried to harm her fetus. Then her fetus got the attention she did not.

Every day in Utah about ten girls between the ages of fifteen and nineteen get pregnant, so let's imagine another poor teen in rural Utah finds herself in a similar situation tomorrow—pregnant with an unhelpful boyfriend, and let's say it's early enough that our hypothetical teen could still legally have an abortion. Legislators intent on ensuring nothing like the case of J.M.S. happens again would pursue two policy goals. The first is state support of the right to parent—creating a climate where women who want to continue pregnancies aren't shamed, forced out of school or employment for lack of day care, or economically unable to parent that child well. The second is state support of the right to not have a child—ensuring easy access to contraception and early access to safe legal abortion for those women who don't want to create or continue pregnancies.

A teen like J.M.S. might want to have a baby, or she (alone or in agreement with her parents) might decide having a baby in her situation with this partner is not in her best interest. But the only place in Utah you can get an abortion for reasons other than medical need, Salt Lake City, is a 3½-hour drive from where J.M.S. lived; it's 7 hours when there's snow in the mountains. Utah law currently requires a 72-hour waiting period after in-person counseling, so she has to find a health care professional in her area to counsel her, or have access to the technology to do it by video with the clinic, or go to the clinic herself. Utah law prohibits Medicaid from paying for "elective" abortion, and private insurance coverage for abortion in Utah is rare, so our hypothetical teen will have to find hundreds of dollars for the procedure itself. (The average cost of a nonhospital first-trimester abortion with local anesthesia at ten weeks is approximately $500.) Raising that fee, plus money to get to Salt Lake City and potentially stay the night in a hotel after the procedure, delays abortion to later gestational ages (assuming she can raise this money at all). There's no public transportation where J.M.S. lived, so she has to have or borrow a car. The sedation used in many abortion procedures means she must have a person in her life willing to come to the clinic with her to accompany her home afterward. (Utah abortion clinics don't currently have the capacity to provide the abortion pill through telemedicine. This is something that could improve access for rural women, yet 19 states currently prohibit it.) And in Utah, a teenager like J.M.S. can't get an abortion unless a parent consents to it, or she goes through a court proceeding to get a waiver of the parental consent requirement from a judge.

So is the J.M.S. story about abortion access? Amazingly, according to one newspaper report she made it to an abortion clinic, but not in time—she was told she was too far along to end her pregnancy. What does the word "legal" mean when it is this difficult to exercise that right?

A third response would be to say the J.M.S. story is about preventing unwanted pregnancy, and that looking forward means reducing unwanted teen pregnancies in the first place. But Utah law doesn't allow health teachers to "advocate or encourage" the use of contraception. Three days after the Utah legislature amended the homicide law in response to the J.M.S. case, a bill that would change that stance, allowing comprehensive sex education for students who have parental permission to receive it, lacked support and died in the Education Committee.

A fourth response would be that the J.M.S. story is about her larger economic and social context. A reproductive justice perspective would consider the technological "fix" of contraception and abortion as a necessary but insufficient response. It would go on to an analysis of economic justice, which reminds us that women also need the kind of education, job opportunity, and strong personal and community support that allow everyone to flourish, and reduce the odds of a situation like this ever arising in the first place.

***

Thinking back to the cases discussed in Chapter 2 shows that the Supreme Court struggles with abortion vocabulary too. In *Roe, Casey,* and *Carhart* three seemingly simple words suddenly become complex: "mother," "late," and "birth."

Mother: Earlier I asked what word we should use for the entity in the uterus. The three Supreme Court opinions discussed in Chapter 2 prompt a parallel question: what should we call the person carrying it? "The pregnant woman" is the term generally used by the *Roe* majority, and "the woman" is the term generally used by the *Casey* plurality. In contrast, the *Carhart* majority calls her "the expectant mother" at one point, and at another point it refers to her as a mother even after she has terminated her pregnancy. ("It is self-evident that a mother who comes to regret her choice to abort. . . .") The federal statute *Carhart* reviewed uses "mother" throughout to describe a woman having an abortion. In *Roe,* Justice White's dissenting opinion calls her "the mother" or "the pregnant mother."

When does a woman become a mother? Is it the day she conceives, or the day she delivers? How about the day she is sure she will continue the pregnancy to delivery? The day the fetus is viable? (Interestingly, both the *Roe* and *Casey* majority opinions switch to the term "the mother" when discussing post-viability abortions allowed for life and health.) Or should we give up looking for a fixed social definition of when a woman becomes a mother, and defer to what each person decides for herself? Imagine two pregnant women: one is thrilled and refers to herself as a mother after her first positive pregnancy test; the second plans to terminate or to give the baby up for adoption and says she was never a mother. Can they both be right?

Pregnant women don't fit the typical dictionary definition of "mother": "a woman in relation to a child or children to whom she has given birth." But pregnancy is a liminal state that puts women betwixt and between, and in the second trimester, visibly changed bodies begin marking pregnant women as different from most other people on the street. Transitional states are stressful, so the urge to push people into concrete categories is understandable: shall we keep her in "woman," meaning her pregnancy doesn't change her identity unless and until she delivers, or push her to "mother," meaning her pregnancy immediately put her into another familiar status? (One could argue that the word "mother" doesn't preclude "woman," but it does subsume it. I am both a woman and a wife, but calling me "the wife" reduces my individual identity to a relational identity in a way "the married woman" or "the woman" does not.)

I reject the term "mother" for women seeking abortion because it imposes a role these women are actively rejecting or postponing, and it subtly asserts that a fetus has the same moral status as a child. When I'm speaking for myself, I'm likely to say "woman." When I'm teaching or speaking to a broad audience, I try to respect the tension of the transitional state by using the term "pregnant woman."

Late: *Carhart* uses "late-term" several times to describe second-trimester abortions. (Similarly, advocates and newspapers describe recent proposals to ban abortion at 20 weeks as banning "late abortion.") Because a baby born at 40 weeks is born "at term," and because second-trimester abortions happen in the middle trimester of pregnancy, an obvious description would be "midterm." But pro-fetal rights advocates battle for the American imagination by recasting pre-viability abortions at 13–24 weeks (the second trimester) as "late" or "late-term."

The word "late" has negative personal connotations, as in "tardy." In the context of "choice," a person who is "late" has missed the deadline for a decision. The word recasts women seeking "late abortions" as either having missed the window of opportunity for deciding, or as asking for an exceptional thing that is in our power to grant or deny. Yet since 1973 the legal deadline for abortion has been viability (which is now approximately 24 weeks), so women having abortions in the second trimester are not late in this sense.

Alternatively, the word "late" could be defended as referring to the last portion of the approximately 24-week window in which people have a constitutional right to terminate pregnancy. But combining "late" with "term" ("late-term abortions") makes a conceptual switch. Pregnancy doesn't end at 24 weeks; babies "carried to term" are born at approximately 40 weeks.* Adding the word "term" puts abortion timing in the context of pregnancy as a whole, so "late-term abortion" subtly suggests a fetus close to healthy delivery—or, at minimum, one that is viable.

That's why terms like "late abortion" and "late-term abortion" don't seem like fair or accurate synonyms for second-trimester abortions. It makes more sense to call abortions that occur before the constitutional deadline of viability "early" (first trimester; 1–12 weeks) and "midterm" (second trimester; 13–24 weeks), and the rare ones that really do occur in the third trimester "late" (e.g., post-viability abortions done because the woman's life or health is threatened, or nonviable fetuses aborted after 24 weeks). To say proposals to ban

* Ironically, a recent government poster designed to educate pregnant women is titled "Pregnancy: Know Your Terms." It tells them "Early Term" is 37 weeks through 38 weeks and 6 days, "Full Term" is 39 weeks through 40 weeks and 6 days, and "Late Term" is 41 weeks to 41 weeks and 6 days. No wonder the idea of a "late-term abortion" triggers revulsion! NIH National Child and Maternal Health Education Program, https://www.nichd.nih.gov/ncmhep/initiatives/know-your-terms/pages/materials.aspx [accessed Apr. 2, 2017]. See also, Spong CY. Defining "term" pregnancy: recommendations from the Defining "Term" Pregnancy Workgroup. *JAMA*. 2013;309:2445–2446.

abortion after 20 weeks address "midterm abortions" is not to say whether these bans are good or bad. It accurately identifies the fact they target the middle of pregnancy.

Birth: The federal statute considered in *Carhart* calls the banned procedure "partial birth abortion." "Partial birth" was used to describe moving part of a nonviable fetus out of the uterus into the vaginal canal. But "birth" is the process by which a living baby leaves a woman's body. The words "birth" and "abortion" are contradictory, but by inventing a term that combined them, opponents of the procedure successfully conjured images of infanticide. That was their goal: the Congressional Findings preceding the bill say the procedure has a "disturbing similarity to the killing of a newborn infant," that banning it will "draw a bright line that clearly distinguishes abortion and infanticide," and that allowing it "will further coarsen society to the humanity of not only newborns, but all vulnerable and innocent human life, making it increasingly difficult to protect such life."

Could the "partial birth abortion" controversy constitute a moral panic? Banning the procedure didn't prevent any pregnancies from being terminated. As Congress intended, doctors continued to do what they did before this new method was developed: they use traditional dilation and extraction (D&E) in the second trimester. Unlike the intact version (which was dubbed "partial birth"), traditional D&E dismembers a fetus in the uterus before it is removed. Many might find the medical facts of that procedure just as objectionable, but abortion is a constitutional right before approximately 24 weeks (viability) and those are the only options—the nonviable fetus will be removed either intact or not intact. Second-trimester terminations represent only one-tenth of all American abortions (the most recent statistics are that 10% are between 13 and 20 weeks, and 1.3% are at 21 weeks or later), and most of them did not use the controversial intact D&E method. (There was no data on exactly how many abortions were done using that procedure, but researchers at the Guttmacher Institute estimated that in 2000 it was approximately 0.17% of all abortions.)

Yet efforts to ban the procedure generated a firestorm of legislation, litigation, and media reports. Congress passed bans on the procedure in 1996 and 1997, but President Clinton vetoed them both. By 2000, about 30 states had banned the procedure. A challenge to Nebraska's ban made it to the U.S. Supreme Court, which struck down Nebraska's law against intact D&Es because its inclusion of traditional D&Es made it an undue burden on the abortion right and it didn't include the required exception for the health of the woman (*Stenberg v. Carhart,* 2000). Then Congress went back to the drawing board, passing a revised ban that was more specific and included an exception for when a woman's life is threatened (though not when her health is threatened). That law was signed by President Bush and approved by the Supreme Court in *Gonzales v. Carhart* in 2007.

Why did this procedure capture so much attention? Second-trimester fetuses can't survive outside the womb, but linking type of abortion and infanticide may have made the procedure represent "abortion out of control." A moral panic typically has three elements, and these elements—exaggeration and distortion (equating the legal abortion of nonviable fetuses with infanticide), prediction (the claim this procedure could later lead to actual infanticide), and symbolization (a rarely used procedure comes to represent all abortion)—all seem to be there.

* * *

Indulge me: If you think abortion should be legal one week into pregnancy, put your hand up. Now, if you think abortion should not be legal one week before full-term delivery, put that hand back down.

If you didn't raise your hand at all, that means you think abortion *should* be illegal one week into pregnancy. If that's your view, now it's your turn—please put your hand up. Now, do you think that a law banning abortion should include any exceptions? (Making abortion legal in cases of rape, or incest, or when a woman's life or health is threatened by pregnancy, or when the fetus has a serious anomaly, or anything else you like.) If yes, you think a general ban on abortion should have one or more exceptions, put that hand back down.

If your hand went up and down, you have a mixed position. If it moved in response to the first paragraph, you're pro-choice for women in early pregnancy, and pro-fetal rights for women in late pregnancy. If it moved in response to the second paragraph, you're pro-choice for whatever women are described by the exception(s) you chose (survivors of rape or incest, etc.—you're not saying they *must* get abortions, only that the choice is up to them), and pro-fetal rights for all other women.

For people with mixed positions like these, terms like "pro-life" and "pro-choice" are inaccurate and incomplete. I've done this experiment with several lecture halls full of people, and if they turn out to be representative, "mixed position" would be the label for the vast majority of Americans.

Yet in a 2015 Gallup poll asking Americans if they were pro-life or pro-choice, only 3% reported "mixed position or neither."

My friend Betty described herself as pro-life for most of her forty-something years. When she became accidentally pregnant in college she immediately knew she'd deliver and raise that baby, and her family life has been a tremendous joy to her ever since. She jokes that she lives in "one of the last Catholic ghettos in the U.S.," and she loves being an extremely active member of her church.

Yet recently, her views on abortion shifted. A family member in a sad medical situation had an abortion, and that made Betty wonder: If abortion is okay for her, why isn't it okay for other people? Her teenage son made the startling declaration that he was pro-choice. ("Mom! It's the only position that makes sense!") I asked for her feedback on an early draft of the Introduction to this book. A freelance job brought her to the 2017 Chicago Women's March, and some of the speakers she heard that day made sense to her.

Then it happened: in a Chicago grocery store she saw a young woman wearing a t-shirt that said, "This Is What An ABORTION ACCESS SUPPORTER Looks Like."

"And I was like, that's it! That's me!" Betty told me. "I'm not for abortion. I honestly wish all undesired pregnancies were stopped before conception. But I am for abortion access."

Betty approached the stranger and put her hand up. "High five on the shirt!" The surprised young woman slapped her hand and said thanks, mentioning that she'd gotten a lot of scornful looks for it in their neighborhood, and they parted.

Betty pushed her cart up the ice cream aisle. "Huh," she thought. "I guess I'm pro-choice."

Words matter. They're powerful, so we should be thoughtful about our word choice. That doesn't mean we should be precious or fearful about it. When someone uses a term you don't care for, be generous and curious: tell me more about that word, what does it mean to you? "Diversity" usually refers to identities like race, ethnicity, gender, sexual orientation, and religion. But the philosophical diversity of Americans is part of our national character as well.

So why don't we set aside the labels for a moment, acknowledge that abortion has been a constitutional right for 45 years, and move on to a richer conversation about ethics?

Chapter 4

Abortion Ethics I

Whether

When I was a child, I loved scrambling through a gigantic, anatomically correct heart and watching newborn chicks peck out of their shells at Chicago's Museum of Science and Industry. But I was most captivated by the museum's collection of human embryos and fetuses—twenty-four jars showing human development between 4 weeks (a tiny speck lit from behind) to almost 38 weeks (a fully formed baby on the cusp of delivery). As a child I returned to this display again and again, mesmerized by the secrets it revealed.

Yet other things are obscured by clear glass. The last time I was at the museum I was 41 weeks pregnant, my hands resting on my giant belly as I tried to waddle myself into labor. Where was I in this display, where was my body? In a macabre flight of fantasy, I imagined what it would look like if instead of miscarrying, the twenty-four pregnant women who donated these specimens also died, and the display presented their cadavers with their bellies dissected open. How would exhibiting these embryos and fetuses in their original "containers" change the story of human development this exhibit told? Today sonograms are our jars—to show us what's inside the womb, they also must erase women's bodies from our field of vision.

We can see a woman, or we can see her embryo or fetus, but we can't see both simultaneously.

This visual swing between women and the embryos or fetuses living inside them reminds me of the famous optical illusion merging an old and young woman in one drawing. Our eyes can switch between seeing one or the other with utter clarity, and intellectually you know they're both there, but it's almost impossible to focus on both simultaneously. Abortion ethics wrestles with the same issue of dual focus. Autonomy approaches often focus on women, and biological approaches focus on embryos or fetuses. Relational and multi-criterion approaches, which consider multiple parties and multiple principles, better fit what some people experience as everyday moral reasoning, but are harder to implement as a matter of policy. And one of the most familiar policy arguments in favor of legal abortion—that women will suffer great harm if it's illegal—is rooted in the consequentialist calculus of public health ethics.

So which of these approaches to abortion ethics is right? Is abortion ethical, or isn't it?

Several years ago I had lunch with Sidney and Dan Callahan, an engaging couple that has written about abortion both together and separately. Sidney is pro-life, and she provided some of the first arguments for a group she belongs to called Feminists for Life. Dan is a prominent bioethicist who is pro-choice, and his first book on abortion was cited by the Supreme Court in *Roe v Wade*. After lunch Sidney invited me back to her house to talk further. She's a smart, warm woman with a silver bob, six children, and a Ph.D. in psychology, and I felt right at home in her living room filled with bookshelves, art, and Oriental rugs.

"Pro-life people believe there is a moral reality," Sidney explained. She thinks the probabilities are higher than not that her analysis of the moral status of embryos and fetuses is true—high enough to base law on it. I asked her to imagine a person who shared her views of embryos and fetuses, but didn't agree with her view that birth control is morally permissible. If this person wanted to make birth control illegal because it also interrupts the procreative process, how would she respond? Sidney said that person is wrong—they haven't persuaded her, and birth control should be a matter of conscience. Why isn't the same true for abortion? Because the abortion line is right, she said.

There are strong ethical arguments for and against abortion throughout pregnancy. That fact helps to explain why forty-five years of argument haven't brought consensus on the moral status of embryos and fetuses. I interpret the never-ending debate on abortion as a different kind of consensus: confirmation that the moral status of embryos and fetuses cannot be proven to the degree necessary to justify government imposition of a single view.

Abortion is a matter of the heart. That's why abortion decisions in our secular, pluralistic society must be left to individual conscience. Some people think Sidney is wrong about abortion—her intellectual arguments for pro-life feminism haven't persuaded them, and their intellectual arguments for pro-choice feminism haven't persuaded her. I respect her strong feeling that she "just knows" the high moral status of embryos and fetuses. But in a pluralistic society, that's not sufficient justification for one group to impose its vision on others by force of law.

Roe v. Wade was premised on a lack of consensus. The *Roe* Court was wise to conclude that "[w]hen those trained in the respective disciplines of medicine, philosophy, and theology are unable to arrive at consensus" "on when life begins," the Constitution prohibits government from either requiring or prohibiting abortion. Forty-five years later, those "trained in medicine, philosophy, and theology"—who today include bioethicists—still haven't reached consensus. Framing lack of consensus as consensus of a different sort may be as frustrating as it is liberating, but living with disagreement is both the price and pleasure of pluralism.

Some argue that if we're uncertain about the moral status of embryos and fetuses, we should err on the side of prohibiting their destruction. However, as the chapter on abortion storytelling helps to illustrate, what we have now isn't uncertainty, it's disagreement. Some Americans are very certain embryos and fetuses have full moral status from the moment of conception. (The bumper sticker summary? "It's a Child, Not a Choice.") Others are very certain embryos and fetuses have little or no moral status until later stages, up to and including delivery. (The bumper sticker summary? "It's not a chicken. It's an egg.") A third group believes that moral status is conferred socially. This camp would say a woman who aborts at 6 weeks without guilt, and a woman who mourns a miscarriage at 6 weeks the same as a newborn's death, are both correct. (The bumper sticker summary? "Trust Women.") And of course some of us are just plain uncertain. But to say "we" are uncertain about the moral status of embryos and fetuses is inaccurate. We disagree about it.

Our disagreement is why *Roe* protected pluralism. As the Supreme Court put it in *Casey*, the 1992 case that affirmed *Roe*:

> Men and women of good conscience can disagree, and we suppose some always shall disagree, about the profound moral and spiritual implications of terminating a pregnancy, even in its earliest stage. Some of us as individuals find abortion offensive to our most basic principles of morality, but that cannot control our decision. Our obligation is to define the liberty of all, not to mandate our own moral code. … At the heart of liberty is the right to define one's own concept of existence, of meaning, of the universe, and of the mystery of human life. The underlying constitutional issue is whether the State can resolve these philosophic questions in such a definitive way that a woman lacks all choice in the matter… .

Disagreement can include uncertainty. (It's fair to say all assessments of embryos and fetuses include some degree of uncertainty, since none can be proven indisputably correct.) But in the modern history of the United States, disagreement and uncertainty on moral issues leads to legal freedom, not legal demands. Where there's strong moral consensus (e.g., the immorality of killing an adult), the collective is entitled to dictate behavior and to expect lawbreakers to be punished. Where there's disagreement (e.g., the immorality of killing animals), a pluralistic society allows people to make their own choices, and expects vegetarians and carnivores to peacefully coexist.

The argument from uncertainty also fails to address the moral status of women, about which we are certain: 100% people. The fetal rights version of the argument from uncertainty says, "In an area of so much uncertainty, and with such high negative consequences for the potential person (death of this embryo or fetus), we should err on the side of life." Including women in the analysis flips the weight of uncertainty in support of pluralism rather than abortion bans: "In an area of so much uncertainty, and with such high negative consequences for the uncontested person (an unwanted pregnancy), we should err on the side of her life and moral judgment."

Roe and *Casey* do not say that embryos and fetuses have no moral status before viability. They say they have no legal status under the Constitution. According to the *Roe* Court, that's because the original intent of those who wrote the Constitution did not encompass embryos and fetuses in the word "person." The fact that there is no secular proof or reasoning that would support a re-interpretation of the Constitution's use of the word "person" to include embryos and fetuses is what keeps it that way. In contrast, women are "persons" protected by the Constitution.

I respect the intelligence and goodwill of those who feel intense empathy toward, and responsibility for, embryos and fetuses. Pluralism is why I embrace honest abolitionists who oppose abortion—I want to understand these neighbors better, and to find ways to work together. And pluralism is why I'm willing to fight those who oppose abortion's legality—I want to protect other neighbors from losing the right to make this critical decision according to their own conscience. If we were all more specific about exactly what we oppose and support, perhaps our conversations would be more precise and productive.

My lunch companion's experience of "just knowing" is the definition of faith, and pluralism is one reason American constitutional law also respects others who "just know" otherwise. Abortion was correctly identified as a constitutionally protected right, and it must remain legal. That's not negotiable for me.

Do you remember the grid I introduced in Chapter 1, separating the analysis of the constitutional status of abortion from the analysis of the ethics of abortion? Let's leave the law behind for a moment and focus on that second column, because I am also convinced that the ethics of abortion is a question about which reasonable people can disagree. The moral worth of embryos and fetuses can't be proven by science; it springs from belief. What do you believe, and why?

Disagreement about the ethics of abortion doesn't have to threaten the legal right to abortion. Reviewing many abortion arguments leading to different conclusions (as well as those that reach the same conclusion through different reasoning) explains one reason our culture continues to struggle with abortion. They all have their strengths—stare at any approach to abortion ethics long enough and you'll be temporarily convinced. Considering them together is like reading a comparative religion text reviewing the beauties of different faith traditions. Both remind me why these are matters of conscience, not state policy. These ethical arguments also point out that a common impression—that arguments against abortion are about ethics, and arguments for abortion are only about law or policy—is incorrect.

The moral seriousness (or lack thereof) of ordinary abortion is simmering under the surface of our abortion debate. The vast majority of abortions are not for medical need, and nine out of ten of them happen in the first trimester (89% before 12 weeks LMP; 66% before 8 weeks LMP). Yet the way our public debate revolves around cases of abortions done for extreme medical need, or abortions done in the second trimester, means we don't hear the ethical analysis of the more typical "I'm two months pregnant and I don't want to have a baby"—not now, or not with this guy, or insert-your-ordinary-reason here. All the ethical arguments I review in the following chapters have something to say about ordinary abortion.

There are many ways to think about "the whether question"—whether abortion is ever ethical. In the remainder of this chapter I summarize several approaches to abortion ethics—biological, autonomy, public health, relational (including care and feminist ethics), and multi-factorial—that cover most of the common arguments in abortion ethics. In Chapter 5 I move on to "the when question": if abortion is ethical at the beginning of pregnancy, when (if ever) as pregnancy advances does it become unethical?

Philosophers might find this chapter too thin (since no summary can do any theory full justice) and non-philosophers might find it too dense (since no summary can turn any theory into beach reading). So I encourage those who want to learn more to dig into the many books and articles that have been written on these approaches and those interested in less detail to aim for comprehension of the general framework. This chapter is meant as a survey giving you a sense of a range of approaches to abortion ethics. It isn't possible to provide a comprehensible summary of every way in the world one could think about abortion ethics in one chapter. If a theory or author you favor isn't identified here, I hope you'll add it to the list in your conversations.

An obvious gap in this review of ethical approaches to abortion is religious reasoning. Different religions have different perspectives on abortion. Within each religion, there are differences between official doctrine and the beliefs or actions of the people in that religion. (For example, Catholic doctrine says abortion is almost always impermissible. However, 38% of Americans who identify themselves as Catholic say abortion is morally acceptable. And 24% of American abortion patients report they are Catholic, which means Catholic women have abortions at about the same rate as the general population. So what exactly is "the Catholic position" on abortion?) That's one reason I won't presume to tell you what your religion's position is on abortion.

My focus in this book is secular ethics—ethical approaches to abortion that don't rely on the existence of a God or a Divine Creator, a belief in one, or acceptance of any particular religion's rules. If your personal morality flows from a religious tradition, you still might see secular reasoning in this chapter that resonates with you, or that reaches a similar conclusion by a different route, or that inspires you to learn more about how your religion's reasoning responds to that argument.

If you've already concluded abortion is obviously and irrefutably ethical or unethical, perhaps this chapter will help you understand how other loving, wise people in your life might see things differently. Earlier I said more private discussion of abortion experience would be productive. Thoughtful conversations about abortion opinion would help as well. So think of this chapter as an invitation to friendly discussion about your thoughts on abortion generally with your family, friends, and neighbors.

1. BIOLOGICAL APPROACHES TO ABORTION ETHICS (DNA/CONCEPTION)

Arguments in this category of the "Whether" question rely on biology, which requires a basic understanding of how pregnancy begins.

An egg ("oocyte") and a sperm ("spermatozoon") are each a single cell that contains 23 chromosomes—half the number found in all other human cells. In a typical month, a woman's ovaries release one egg during ovulation. If the timing of intercourse allows sperm and egg to connect (sperm can survive several days), fertilization occurs in the fallopian tube. A sperm breaks the egg's membrane, enters it, and releases the sperm's nucleus. When the two nuclei of these single cells fuse, it becomes a new single-celled organism with 46 chromosomes (23 pairs) called a zygote. Then it begins the process of mitosis, where cells double and divide, double and divide. Approximately 12 to 18 hours after fertilization, it's a two-celled zygote; after about 40 hours, it's four cells. After about 80 hours, it's a multi-cell entity called an early morula; after four days, it's called an advanced morula. In the first five days of its existence, it travels down the fallopian tube to the uterus; after five days, it's called a blastocyst. Approximately 6.5 days after fertilization, the blastocyst sinks into the wall of the uterus, which is called implantation. Two weeks after conception, at the start of the third week of its existence, it's called an embryo.

The one-celled zygote contains the genetic blueprint for a human being. One argument calls this "substantial identity." According to this view, people are intrinsically valuable because of what we are, and what we are is a physical organism, which comes to be at conception. After conception we get bigger (quantitative change) but we don't undergo substantial qualitative change through development to an adult human being.

A different argument based on the same fact is sometimes called "potential theory." Potential theory asserts that we should value entities in their transitive state because of their potential to become something else. People with this view don't claim a zygote, morula, blastocyst, or embryo is "substantially" a person; they focus on the fact it could become a person in the future. Because that one-celled entity contains everything necessary to become a person, this potential person should be protected just as actual people are.

One strength of conception arguments is their clarity and simplicity. Before their union, an egg and sperm can never become a person. After their union, they can. Development after conception is a continuous process, and the only other developmental turning point as clear and simple as conception is birth.

Philosopher Don Marquis offers a variation on a biological potential argument that emphasizes experience more than physicality. This is the "value of a future like ours" argument. Marquis argues that the standard arguments for and against abortion that revolve around categorizing fetuses as persons or non-persons miss the essence of the matter, which to him is our shared assumption that killing adults is morally wrong. Why is that true? Because, Marquis says, killing deprives an adult of his or her future—a set of experiences, projects, and activities that this adult will now never have. He argues that every embryo and fetus has a comparable set of experiences, projects, and activities in its future, and the loss of that future is at least as great to an embryo or fetus as the loss of that future is to an adult human being who is killed. Therefore, "since the reason that is sufficient to explain why it is wrong to kill human beings after the time of birth is a reason that also applies to fetuses, it follows that abortion is prima facie seriously morally wrong."

Critique of Biological (DNA/Conception) Approaches to Abortion Ethics

One critique of this approach to abortion ethics says it defies common sense to say people are "substantially" the same as tiny one-celled (or two, or thirty-two, etcetera) creatures. Yes, we share some properties, but qualities like rationality aren't just "quantitative" changes, they are qualitative changes—essential additional properties we gain long after conception that are of great moral significance.

Another critique is it's scientifically flawed. It's not true that a fertilized egg (or a blastocyst or an embryo) contains "everything it needs" to become a person. A second condition necessary to its becoming a person is it has to live inside a woman's body. (When one of these entities is frozen and stored in a fertility clinic, this reality becomes quite clear.) So to separate the analysis of fertilized eggs from the female bodies by which they must be nourished for many months contradicts the biological reality in which a DNA approach purports to be grounded.

A relational version of the scientific critique would point out that the woman in whom the embryo or fetus lives is virtually absent in Marquis's "value of a future like ours" argument. Therefore, it fails to account for the embryo or fetus's unique physical dependency, or what sustaining another life costs a woman physically, socially, emotionally, and financially. One could argue that these differences are significant enough to undermine Marquis's conclusion that pregnant women and their fetuses stand in the same moral relationship as adult murderers and their adult victims.

Writer Katha Pollitt analyzes the biological argument from a practical angle. In *Pro: Reclaiming Abortion Rights*, she observes that about half of all fertilized eggs fail to implant and are washed out with menstrual flow. After implantation, 10–20% of known pregnancies end in miscarriages. So if fertilized eggs are morally equivalent to born people (either because of their DNA or because of their potentiality), why aren't we devoting tremendous research dollars to stopping miscarriage? To Pollitt, the fact that those who say personhood begins at conception aren't also upset about the natural, yet still epidemic, level of miscarriage suggests they are more intent on controlling women than rescuing zygotes, blastocysts and embryos. Conceptually, Pollitt sees DNA in this context as a secular synonym for the religious idea of ensoulment.

I am moved by potentiality, but that is different than being bound by it. We can be awed by the fact a tiny acorn might someday provide shade, while still acknowledging that acorns planted in my yard don't have the same value as mature oak trees.

2. AUTONOMY APPROACHES TO ABORTION ETHICS

Autonomy arguments focus on adults as individuals. Modern medical ethics presumes that patients are moral agents who can and should decide what happens to and in their own bodies and lives. Autonomy approaches to abortion ethics begin with this widely accepted ethical principle, and argue that pregnancy does not change an adult's right to control her body. In bioethics, autonomy is defined as "personal rule of self that is free from both controlling interferences by others and from personal limitations that prevent meaningful choices, such as inadequate understanding."

The philosophical framework in which autonomy approaches are embedded, which is called principlism, is a large part of what launched the field of medical ethics. This is one appeal of autonomy approaches to abortion ethics—the fact they are grounded in this history. Medical ethicists and patients rejected the earlier "doctor knows best" model of paternalism, because only patients can filter medical facts and recommendations through their own personal values to make final decisions.

Autonomy ethics are also familiar because they are consistent with, and have been incorporated into, American law. For example, patient autonomy creates an ethical duty for physicians to obtain a patient's informed consent before treating them, and now the law also requires this. Our familiarity with laws grounded in autonomy sometimes makes us forget they are also (and often started as) ethical principles. That contributes to the false impression that prochoice arguments grounded in autonomy are only about law. As Ann

Furedi, the chief executive of a British not-for-profit provider of abortion services, puts it in *The Moral Case for Abortion*: pro-choice isn't "informed indifference," it's a judgment that "the right to make one's own choices should be valued in its own right and judged to be important in itself."

Another appeal of autonomy approaches is they are relatively straightforward. They identify (and justify) the decisionmaker, and avoid altogether the content or outcome of the decision. Autonomy approaches say individual dignity cannot flourish unless the person who will be most affected by a decision retains the authority to make that decision for themselves. It doesn't say all options are equal; it says whatever arguments can be made for or against a particular set of options do not outweigh this value of decisionmaking authority. The principle of autonomy says nothing about whether the best response to your cancer is palliative care or aggressive experimental treatment; it says only that the decision should be up to you. The same is true for abortion: the principle of autonomy says nothing about whether the best response to your unwanted pregnancy is continuing or ending it; it says only that the decision should be up to you.

The traditional approach to autonomy assumes one patient, and designates patients with capacity as decisionmakers. When applied to abortion ethics, it does the same. It could be said to ignore embryos and fetuses, or it could be said to treat them with what's essentially a jurisdictional assessment: you own your body, and therefore as long as an embryo or fetus is located inside your body, your values dictate what happens with it too. A biological addendum to this "jurisdictional approach" would argue that because embryos and fetuses can't be physically autonomous before viability (they die if taken outside a woman's body), the principle of autonomy cannot be applied to them at all.

Some arguments against abortion focus on embryonic or fetal potential. The traditional autonomy approach can be seen as focusing on adult potential—the life a woman can have when she's able to control her reproduction as she sees fit. Autonomy theories consider adults as having lives still in the process of unfolding. Like any adult confronting a life-altering body change he or she doesn't want, autonomy theories applied to abortion give great moral weight to the potential that's lost if a woman decides this pregnancy and/or parenting will curtail her future.

A second autonomy approach to abortion ethics grants the possibility of embryonic or fetal personhood and assumes two people. It observes that American adults are never required to sacrifice their bodies to save another person, and argues there's no reason pregnant women should be held to a different standard.

The most famous of these arguments was made by philosopher Judith Jarvis Thomson in 1971. She posited a parallel universe in which you wake up to find an adult, who happens to be a violinist, is attached to your body. He needs to be plugged into your circulatory system in order to live, and if you disconnect him he will die. She argues that the adult violinist has a right to life, but that is different than having a right to *life support* from another person's body. According to Jarvis Thomson, a right to life is a right not to be killed—so if the violinist was flourishing on his own, shooting him at his recital would violate his right to life. But the violinist's right to life does not include a right to be kept alive—so if he needs your body to stay alive, it is not unethical for you to disconnect him. Sacrificing your body to keep someone alive makes you a Good Samaritan, but it's not morally required. This leads Jarvis Thomson to reason that even if an embryo or fetus has the same moral value as an adult, abortion is morally permissible.

No one has ever woken up attached to a violinist. However, three real situations in which the actions of one person involve death or harm to another person support two-person autonomy arguments about abortion like Jarvis Thomson's: organ donation, self-defense, and slavery.

Organ donation is not called "the obligation of life." It's called "the gift of life" because American medical ethics and law both say that no person can be forced to give a piece of their body to another. Our commitment to bodily integrity is so strong that we respect your wishes even after you're dead—your desire to be buried intact is valued more in our culture than another person's desire to stay alive. This rule remains true even if a member of your family, including your child, will die without your help. You are allowed to say, "I don't love you enough," or "I don't know you well enough to want to save you," or "I'm scared."

For example, Robert McFall suffered from a rare bone disease, but the only suitable donor he could find, his cousin David Shimp, refused to donate his bone marrow. McFall asked a court to order his cousin to save his life, and the court refused. McFall died three weeks later. The court reasoned that Shimp's refusal to donate was

> morally indefensible. [But for] our law to *compel* defendant to submit to an intrusion of his body would change every concept and principle upon which our society is founded. ... For a society which respects the rights of one individual, to sink its teeth into the jugular vein or neck of one of its members and suck from it sustenance for another member, is revolting to our hard-wrought concepts of jurisprudence.

Pregnancy can be viewed as a form of organ donation. A woman undergoes significant physical changes that can range from uncomfortable to dangerous for months so another's life can be sustained by her major organs. It occupies her uterus, her heart must pump extra blood to give it oxygen, her kidneys must process its urine, and so on. These similarities mean the choice to lend one's body to a developing human should also be considered a gift, not a requirement.

The American tradition and law of self-defense offers another real-world analogy. When a person breaks into your house, you're allowed to kill him. (The legal standard usually requires imminent threat of serious harm.) This suggests a woman who experiences an unwelcome pregnancy as bodily break-in by a different type of intruder should be able to respond to the threat of physical harm to her body and irrevocable disruption of her life by taking lethal action.

Slavery provides a third analogy. Some opponents of legal abortion have compared it to slavery, arguing that American law used to wrongly define slaves as less than people, and today the same is happening to fetuses. A different way to look at this analogy focuses on actual practice: slavery is a set of laws that force the enslaved to devote his or her body to another person against his or her will. Abortion bans force women with unwanted pregnancies to devote their bodies to another person (an embryo or a fetus, if law defines them as persons) against their will. Therefore, abortion bans should be considered a form of slavery that's also morally abhorrent.*

Dr. Willie Parker adds a personal angle to the last analogy from his perspective as an abortion provider working in the South:

> [I]t is impossible not to think constantly about the analogy of the limits on women's reproductive rights to slavery. As an African American man descended from slaves and raised in the South, it is too easy for me to imagine what it's like to have no control over your body, your destiny, your life. … White men maintained jurisdiction over black women's bodies, in that they owned them and took possession of their babies. Insofar

* Some might argue it's nature that commandeers a woman's body during pregnancy, not the government. But when the force of law is all that's stopping a pregnant woman from using a safe and simple medical intervention to free herself from this unwanted servitude, the government is now what's commandeered her body for the benefit of what the government has deemed "another person."

> as abortion access is limited, this abuse of power extends to all women. I believe that the men who are passing the laws that limit medication abortion want to control women's bodies, which is not so far from wanting to own them outright.

We've reviewed the traditional autonomy approach, which says abortion decisions should be treated like all other medical decisions in which individual adults control their bodies, and an autonomy approach that grants the possibility of two people but concludes physically hosting a second person is a gift rather than an obligation. A third autonomy approach focuses on equity.

An equity of autonomy approach to abortion ethics also grants personhood to two people, but instead of a woman in relation to an embryo or fetus, it would consider the relative autonomy of the man and woman who created the pregnancy together. Two people have sex, but only one becomes pregnant. That is not equitable. However, because the simple medical intervention of safe abortion can remedy this biological imbalance, equity of autonomy means women must be allowed to escape pregnancy's physical risk and impact when they don't see its outcome as a benefit. In other words: Nature isn't fair, but culture can be.

The social impact of parenting can also factor into an equity of autonomy analysis. Arguments focused on embryonic potential turn on the fact an embryo ultimately becomes a child. An equity of autonomy argument takes that point a step further: yes, it will be a child, whom someone will have to take care of. Pregnancy is a diagnosis, and how much time, emotional energy, and money a woman will have to spend raising her child is part of the prognosis. When asked their reasons for abortion, 48% of patients said they didn't want to be a single parent or they were having problems with their husband or partner. So for some women, the parenting contribution the man she created the pregnancy with will or won't make, or what role she does or doesn't want him to play, is an important factor in deciding whether to continue or end an accidental pregnancy.

Pregnant women do not have to parent. Yet few choose to deliver babies for adoption. Statistics are hard to come by, but between 1996 and 2002, only 1% of babies born to single women in the United States were relinquished for adoption in the first month of the baby's life. Another statistic comes from the Turnaway Study, which was mentioned in Chapter 2. This study also analyzed a group of 231 women who came to an abortion facility to end their pregnancy, and were "turned away" because they were beyond that facility's gestational limit. Seventy of the "turn away" women later had an abortion at a different facility, or miscarried. What I find fascinating is that of the 161 who later delivered babies, only 15 (9%) of these women who sought an abortion later chose adoption. Why the vast majority of women prefer either abortion or parenting to adoption is something I hope to explore in future work. Here I simply observe that although the law does not require it, current practice means that for women, continuing a pregnancy is almost synonymous with becoming a parent.

A different version of an "equity of autonomy" approach is offered by philosopher John Rawls. He is also concerned with equality, and he offers a way to think about justice that is as simple as it is powerful: The Veil of Ignorance. Rawls says that to identify the best organizing principles for your society, you should blind yourself to your actual social status and circumstance, then consider institutional structures or constitutional principles from behind a Veil of Ignorance—a place in which you have no idea what role you'll have or play in this society (gender, race, religion, age, disability status, economic status, nationality, and so on). Now ask yourself: what does a just, equitable, or fair arrangement look like? This strategy tries to harness self-interest as an engine for justice. Rawls's argument is that the definition of a just society is one in which we'd all be willing to play any part we were assigned by the roll of the dice. (It also reminds us that our current gender, race, etcetera, is, like a roll of the dice, also a matter of chance.) Rawls assumes that from behind the Veil, we'd all pick the value of equality—and when equality is impossible, that we'd choose inequalities that maximize the benefits of those who are worst off.

Some argue the Veil of Ignorance approach potentially concludes abortion is unjust. Behind the Veil of Ignorance, you must consider the possibility you could be an embryo or fetus instead of the adult you are now. And when you think that's possible, the argument goes, self-interest leads you to favor a world in which embryos and fetuses have a right to life equal to adults, because they are future rights-claimers in society, and you wouldn't want to be aborted.

Behind the Veil of Ignorance, you must also consider the possibility you could be a woman with an unwanted pregnancy. However, those who make the argument above would likely respond that on balance, people would rather risk the harm of life with an unwanted pregnancy over the harm of never enjoying life at all because you were aborted.

Rawls wants us to imagine away all personal ties, because he thinks that objective rationality is the only way to pick concepts of justice. But I will go against his wishes for an abstract "other" rather than a concrete one for a moment, to suggest an amendment: imagine you draw the role of embryo or fetus, so it is your life on the line. But you don't live in the body of some random, faceless lady. You peeked outside the Veil of Ignorance and saw that the woman in whom you live, the woman who rolled "unwanted pregnancy" on the dice, is your actual mother.

My parents moved from Colorado to Indiana the summer after my dad got his Ph.D. He started his new job as an anthropology professor in August, and I was born in October. I'm lucky to have had a wonderful life. I'm as happy as anyone can be to have been born, and

I hope to continue loving and engaging with my family, friends, work, and world for many more decades. But what if the pregnancy that ended in me had been an accident, and my mom was beside herself about it? It's too soon, she's not sure their marriage will survive this stressful time, they'd barely have a single paycheck in the bank when the baby came, she doesn't know anyone in Indiana, and she wanted to finish her education before she started having kids? Would I say, peeking out from behind the Veil, that my life is more important than my mother's? I would not. The fact that I'm grateful to the woman who brought me to life suggests a gift. If she owed me life, I would not be indebted.

It's not a lack of self-esteem that leads me to say my life isn't more important than my mother's—I find me delightful. You know who else is? My sister, born 18 months later. That pattern makes me think a third pregnancy between my mother and father would've also resulted in a terrific person. My parents never had that third pregnancy. But if the embryo that turned into me had been terminated, the fact they wanted two children means my sister would probably now be the older sibling of a person who in the current version of the world was never created. So in foreclosing the possibility of abortion in a "just society" in the scenario in which I'm the embryo of an unwanted pregnancy, I have just harmed my mother, and eliminated the potential life of a third child. It seems narcissistic to say my potential life is more important than my mother's existing life and that third child's potential life.

Picturing myself as an embryo or fetus for whom I'm speaking now, which is what's asked by the Veil of Ignorance, is not the same as imagining being killed as an adult. It's to imagine myself a creature with no awareness of present, past, or future, and no knowledge of possibility or people. So from behind the Veil of Ignorance, for the sake of my mother and the equal potential of that nonexistent third sibling, I would conclude a world in which my embryonic self is terminated is not unjust.

Now go back behind the Veil, and return to Rawls's direction to imagine an abstract "other" rather than your mother. The dice have been rolled again, and your roll could land on "embryo." Can you extend the empathy you might have for your own mother to the random person who just rolled "woman with an unwanted pregnancy"?

Critique of Autonomy Approaches to Abortion Ethics

The traditional bioethics approach to autonomy assumes one patient. One critique is that it masks what some argue is the crux of the abortion debate: whether the embryo or fetus a woman carries has a moral status that means there are two patients in the room. A second critique of the traditional autonomy approach is how its individualistic focus obscures the social determinants of decision-making. For example, to frame a woman aborting because she cannot afford a child, or a couple aborting because they feel unable to raise a child with a disability, as "exercising their autonomy" avoids discussion of what resources society does and does not offer potential parents.

A critique of the autonomy approach that grants embryonic or fetal personhood for the sake of argument invokes a concept that's important across medical ethics: the omission/commission line. In order to continue the life of someone who needs an organ, I have to do something—I have to choose to disrupt my current bodily state to donate. If I refuse and you want to force me, you have to capture me, strap me down, and cut me open against my will. Whether my organ comes out voluntarily or involuntarily, removing it is an act of commission: doing something to the body produces a result.

In contrast, in order to continue the life of an embryo or fetus living inside me, I don't have to do anything—I just have to continue my current bodily state of pregnancy. If I refuse and you want to force me to remain pregnant, you might have to jail me to ensure I won't end it, but you don't have to *invade* my body. Whether my pregnancy continues voluntarily or involuntarily, that's usually considered an act of omission: not doing anything to the body produces a result.

However, if the reason abortion is prohibited is that the law considers the embryo or fetus I carry to be a person, then in a sense "someone" has metaphorically captured me to use my body. Personhood can't be said to justify forcing the continuation of a pregnancy, then disappear in the omission/commission analysis. It's the force of law that makes this tiny thing powerful enough to do the equivalent of strapping an adult down and forcing a bodily invasion.

A second critique of the two-person autonomy approach says the analogy fails on intent. Unlike nefarious adults who enslave people or break into houses, an embryo or fetus has no intent to harm the woman in whom it lives. (This point must be accompanied by a claim that the fetus's intent is the determining factor, not the impact on the person who feels enslaved or broken into.)

And while those harmed by slavers or burglars or violinists are presumed to have done nothing to bring this harm into their lives, adults who consent to sex have taken an action that can bring a pregnancy into their lives. This raises a common claim: Does consent to sex constitute consent to pregnancy and childbirth?

Autonomy: Is a woman's consent to sex consent to pregnancy?

For some, the autonomy argument begins before conception. This perspective says a woman has autonomy in her sexual decisions, but her consent to sex is also her consent to pregnancy and childbearing. (Lack of consent is a common critique of the violinist analogy: a medically needy adult attaching to an unconsenting woman is a defense of abortion after rape, not abortion after consensual sex.)

I'm struck by how much work this argument does. If a woman has *consented* to pregnancy, then we've completely circumvented all conflict over abortion and any guilt about robbing women of autonomy and bodily integrity. (Phew!) The practical problem is the thousands of actual pregnant women saying no. "I didn't consent to pregnancy then, I don't consent to it now, and I want to end it."

A significant amount of the injury and disease doctors treat is preventable, yet I never hear this "implied consent" or "tacit consent" argument raised elsewhere. Everyone knows driving can result in a car crash, but no one argues driving constitutes consent to car crashes and therefore injured drivers shouldn't get medical treatment. This argument doesn't even come up with other unwelcome consequences of sex. (No one calls consent to sex "consent to chlamydia.") Culpability affects sympathy—the man hit out of nowhere while obeying all traffic laws will get more sympathy than the one who foolishly drove in a blizzard, and the man who wore a seatbelt will get more sympathy than the one who didn't. But sympathy is different from treatment. None of these factors will change the medical options available to these drivers. Even a thief shot in the course of a bank robbery still gets treated in the emergency room, with the goal of bringing his body back to baseline.

"Sex is consent to pregnancy and childbirth" only applies to women. Therefore it also fails an equity of autonomy analysis. A man will never become pregnant or deliver a child as a consequence of sex. A woman can come close to his degree of freedom with a safe medical intervention that ends accidental pregnancy. Denying this intervention to women who want it could be justified only by an argument about the proper role of sex or an argument about the moral status of the embryo.

If you think sex is an ordinary activity adults are entitled to engage in for its own sake, you might see pregnancy as a "risk" of sex. This view might make the car accident analogy ring true to you. If you see sex as a sacred act meant primarily for procreation, you might see pregnancy as the purpose of sex. Such a view makes comparing pregnancy to a car accident sound like nonsense. (Assuming you believe your view of sex can and should be imposed on those who view sex differently.) And of course a car crash is always bad—we don't have "wanted" and "unwanted" car accidents—while women's experiences of becoming pregnant can range from the best thing that could happen to them to the worst.

Similarly, your estimate of the moral status of an embryo might play a role. If you think it's zero, or if you think it's high, whether that embryo was created by consensual or nonconsensual sex will probably be irrelevant to you. A person who puts no value on embryos will always approve of abortion, and a person who puts absolute value on them will never approve of abortion. But if you think the moral status of an embryo is intermediate, the moral status of the woman's actions might be something you're inclined to balance against it.

Perhaps this is what leads some to say abortion is acceptable if contraception failed, but not if the couple didn't use contraception at all. This view is a variation on consent: actively trying to prevent pregnancy (with contraception rather than abstinence) means you didn't consent to it, which makes abortion a permissible second step to complete a plan (sex without childbearing) you already formulated and attempted to execute.

The view that consent to sex without contraception is a form of consent to pregnancy could be seen as a more moderate version of "the argument from uncertainty." The argument from uncertainty (discussed at the beginning of this chapter) says if we can't prove the moral status of the embryo, we should err on the side of prohibiting abortion. What I call the "moderate version" of the argument from uncertainty says if we can't prove the moral status of the embryo, we should try to avoid or reduce abortion, using it only to save people from true accidents.

This view judges a large number of women negatively, since two of every five women with unintended pregnancies report they didn't use contraception consistently or at all. In Chapters 1 and 2 I described four women with unwanted pregnancies: two had them after contraceptive failure (Bonnie the graduate student and Martha the mother who had just remarried), and two didn't use contraception (Leslie the graduate student and Amelia the actor). There's no biological difference between these four embryos. And there's no social difference in the distress and disruption an unwanted child would create for all four women. But based on these women's choices at conception, would you withhold treatment for Leslie and Amelia?

The view that consent to sex without contraception is a form of consent to pregnancy also circles back to the question of whose evaluation of moral status counts. What if Leslie and Amelia see the moral status of their embryos, and/or the moral significance of their sexual intent and action, differently from you? Is the evidence for your view strong enough to justify taking their freedom? Or is it sympathy you intend to withhold?

Finally, I wonder if there's overlap between the reasons some women don't use birth control (such as poverty, lack of personal power in their sexual relationship, or being disorganized or a poor planner) and the reasons they decide they aren't in a good position to be parents. Doctors sometimes describe miscarriage as nature's way of screening out pregnancies with biological problems. Dr. David Grimes, a public health advocate discussed below, describes abortion as a social version of miscarriage—screening out pregnancies with economic or interpersonal problems. If lack of contraception is correlated with these problems, some pregnancies that arise from that will fit Grimes's paradigm.

Equity of Autonomy: Is a man's consent to sex consent to fatherhood?

What about men's autonomy? If women get to decide whether or not to be mothers, shouldn't men get to decide whether or not to be fathers?

Most couples agree on how to respond to a pregnancy they've created together. When they disagree, only one person's wishes can prevail. This is an example of "nature isn't fair" for which there is no cultural remedy. (Nature also gives men total autonomy from the burdens of pregnancy and childbirth, another imbalance for which there's no cultural remedy.) It's the woman's body on the line in pregnancy and delivery, not the man's. Therefore, when couples disagree, men aren't allowed to force abortion, and they're not allowed to force childbirth on their unwilling partners. To say a man's consent to sex is his "consent" to biological fatherhood is inaccurate. American law overrides his lack of consent. There's no denying it: when couples disagree, American men lose their reproductive autonomy after sex.

That doesn't explain why a man whose condom broke is stuck paying child support. If we wanted to maximize gender equity where it's possible, we'd change this policy so a man who didn't want to create a child couldn't force the woman to have an abortion, but he also wouldn't be required to support that child. Instead, the collective (i.e., taxpayers) would support the choices of women who continue pregnancy against their male partners' wishes by contributing financial assistance.

Inequity in pregnancy experience and decisionmaking is real. Culture and law can mitigate it in some places, and not others. "You've made your bed . . ." sounds morally tidy. But to say either gender consents to childbearing by consenting to intercourse is a fiction that crumbles under the moral weight it's asked to carry. This returns us to the remaining approaches to the "whether" question of abortion ethics: public health, relational, and multi-factorial.

3. PUBLIC HEALTH APPROACHES TO ABORTION ETHICS

Public health aims to achieve the greatest health benefits for the greatest number of people. What is "health"? There are many definitions, but an enduring one comes from the World Health Organization: "Health is a state of complete physical, mental and social well-being and not merely the absence of disease or infirmity." The breadth of this definition may have been suprising when it was adopted in 1948, but recent definitions of health have followed its spirit, emphasizing not only a healthy body but also high-quality personal relationships, a sense of purpose in life, and self-regard and resilience. Ensuring the conditions for people to be healthy can include a variety of educational, economic, social, and environmental strategies.

Public health ethics is grounded in consequentialism, which judges the rightness of an action by its outcomes. Utilitarianism is a familiar form of consequentialism that specifies happiness as the desired outcome; in public health ethics the value is placed on health. But the public health model of ethical reasoning doesn't just choose the policy that produces the most good and the least harm to health. The goal is to benefit the whole population without knowingly harming individuals or groups. Because this isn't always possible, a central theme of public health ethics is the tension between protecting the health of the population and the rights of specific individuals—for example, when it is and isn't ethical to quarantine someone with multi-drug-resistant tuberculosis who refuses this isolation.

Social justice is a central value in public health ethics. (This priority could be seen as a product of consequentialism, since social status is an important influence on the health of populations.) Therefore, modern public health ethics pays special attention to the interests of powerless or oppressed populations. Modern public health ethics is also associated with a nonjudgmental stance on behavior when such judgment stands in the way of saving lives or preserving health. For example, a public health analysis of a needle exchange program would value reducing blood-borne disease in heroin users over the cost of appearing to condone drug use.

Although policy makers have wrestled for thousands of years with value-laden decisions about protecting the public's health, the concept of "public health ethics" is only a few decades old. Interestingly, public health professionals still rarely characterize their work as having an ethical dimension.

That's true in abortion care as well. For example, Dr. David Grimes is an acclaimed scholar who has worked as an epidemiologist at the Centers for Disease Control and as a gynecologist providing abortions, and he frames his book about the necessity of safe, legal abortion as a "public health story." He doesn't use the term public health ethics, yet much of what he writes in *Every Third Woman In America* uses that analytic approach.

Grimes begins by reviewing the injury and death that occurred when abortion was illegal—the women who died, and the entire wards of hospitals devoted to women battling serious infection. He also points out how poor people and racial minorities were disproportionately burdened. (For example, before abortion was widely legal, hospital committees sometimes approved women for "therapeutic abortion." Grimes cites data showing women in private hospitals were much more likely to be approved than those in municipal hospitals that treated the poor, and white women were more likely to be approved than women of color. And of course affluent white women were more likely than poor or minority women to know of and be able to see private doctors who would secretly do illegal abortions safely.) Then he reviews how the legalization of abortion dramatically reduced death and injury—first by eliminating the danger of clandestine procedures, and then by allowing physicians to openly study and refine procedures to further improve safety—and distributed health benefits more equitably across class and race. He also emphasizes the harm to children associated with unwanted pregnancy, such as preterm birth, child abuse, and poverty.

An argument that legalized abortion preserves women's lives and health and improves their existing children's health is an implied statement of values (that the lives of women and children are more important than embryos and fetuses) and the beginning of a public health ethics argument. Earlier I noted how our familiarity with laws grounded in the ethical principle of autonomy can lead to a false impression that pro-choice arguments are only about law. A failure to articulate the moral underpinning of the familiar "women die when abortion is illegal" public health argument contributes to a similar impression that pro-choice arguments are only about policy, not ethics.

A conceptual switch from restriction to freedom may be another reason public health arguments in favor of abortion access aren't usually framed as "public health ethics" arguments. Public health ethics often focuses on when the health of the population justifies restricting one person's freedom. When is it right to force a business owner who sells dangerous toys to obey a new regulation, or to force quarantine in the tuberculosis example given above? Abortion care works the opposite way: reduced harm and improved health for women and their existing or future children result from giving individuals more freedom, not less.

Yet the public health ethics approach is common in abortion discussion, even if it's rarely labeled as such. Its focus on protecting and enhancing the well-being of populations fits perfectly with the pro-choice focus on the population of women and existing children whose health is protected by avoiding the harms of illegal abortion and the harms of continuing unwanted pregnancy, and enhanced by the economic, social, and health benefits that flow from planning and spacing children. And social justice requires attention to the fact that unintended pregnancy and its harms, and the harms of current laws restricting abortion, still affect poor and minority women disproportionately.

Critique of Public Health Approaches to Abortion Ethics

Public health ethics responds to the physical, psychological, and economic harm women and their existing or future children suffer when abortion is illegal. Yet when a person's action seriously harms another person, arguments about harm to the wrongdoer rarely lead to changes in the law. (Showing me evidence that abusers experience severe depression if they can't batter their wives won't persuade me domestic violence should be legal.) This fact leads us back to the moral status of embryos and fetuses.

Considering embryos and fetuses equivalent to children and adults would obviously alter the utilitarian calculus of "lives saved" by legal abortion. It could be argued that public health approaches to abortion ethics assume that adults and children are members of the community, and embryos and fetuses aren't, while contributing little to nothing to the logic of this premise. I think it's more accurate to say public health approaches to abortion ethics follow the field's recent tradition of non-judgment on behavior, and defer to the pregnant person's liberty to define whether and how embryonic and fetal health should be included in her situation's life-and-health calculus.

One who believes embryos and fetuses are persons could invoke the "restricted liberties" model of public health, prevalent in the 20th-century response to infectious disease, to justify abortion restrictions. If it were established and agreed that an embryo or fetus is a person, one could make a public health ethics argument in favor of restricting the liberty of women carrying them to avoid harm to the health of their embryos or fetuses.

4. RELATIONAL, CARE, AND FEMINIST APPROACHES TO ABORTION ETHICS

Relational, Care, and Feminist approaches to abortion ethics each deserve their own section. However, because they all value lived experience, interactions with others, and embodiment, in the interest of brevity I consider them together.

Relational approaches view personhood as something that's constructed socially, not (or not just) biologically. Relational theories assert that the supposedly autonomous "self" is really shaped by and within both personal and public relationships. Applied to abortion, because relational theories base moral status on membership in social communities and caring relationships, a woman who has a wanted pregnancy and an unwanted pregnancy at two different times in her life is permitted to define the moral status of those two pregnancies differently. This is partly because she is the only person (or certainly the primary one) in relationship with that embryo or fetus, and partly because a large determinant of whether she does or doesn't want a child is the current status of *her* extended web of personal and societal relationships, and the way having a child will or won't change those relationships. Another expression of this approach asserts that because an embryo or fetus is incapable of having a relationship with anyone but the woman in whom it lives, a woman and her pregnancy should be treated as an integrated unit (both physically and morally) that cannot be considered separately.

Lynn Paltrow is the founder of National Advocates for Pregnant Women, a group that advocates for women charged with crimes against the embryo or fetus they carry. She offers a broader type of relational critique, one that exhorts us to expand the web of relationships we consider. When people talk about the ethical duty a woman has to her fetus, Paltrow asks, where is the ethical duty society owes women to provide the education, empowerment, and access necessary to use contraception? To protect her from violence and sexual assault? Where's the duty society owes pregnant women to provide housing, and neighborhoods where the streets are safe enough to use for exercise, and where nutritious food is available? To support education, jobs, and child care so pregnancy never requires the surrender of long-cherished dreams? In a society that seems to feel no moral responsibility to many pregnant women, Paltrow argues it's unjust to turn around and say, "But she's morally responsible to that fetus."

Care ethics builds on the observation that the world is populated by people living in relationships, not people standing alone. Its "ethic of relations" focuses on the need both to fulfill our obligations to others, and to attend to the needs of our relationships themselves (as opposed to only the needs of individual people). This approach began with psychologist Carol Gilligan's research on gender differences in moral reasoning, which documented that in resolution of moral conflict, males are more likely to use a justice perspective that accords with abstract principles, and females are more likely to use a compassion and care perspective that considers context. Nel Noddings then proposed an ethic of care modeled on the maternal perspective. Thinking of care as work or as a practice brings an obvious fact to the foreground: it is impossible to care for everyone. The natural limitation on human time and energy requires everyone to make choices about what relationships they will enter into, and to whom they will devote selfless care. When applied to abortion, this approach weighs the experience and demands of mothering heavily, with regard both to existing children and to a potential future child.

Feminist ethics scrutinizes situations for gender equity, and applying this approach to abortion raises the "equity of autonomy" concept discussed earlier. Feminist ethics defines a woman's freedom to control her reproductive life as a moral imperative because it facilitates her bodily integrity (a value also explored in the autonomy discussion), her sexual autonomy, and her ability to actively choose if, when, and how her expenditure on mothering will occur, all of which are central to her personhood. Women have a moral right to social equality. Therefore they must have reproductive control, which is a prerequisite to the ability to pursue satisfying and profitable employment, and it expands social and political opportunity for women individually and as a group.

Philosopher Susan Sherwin underscores another feminist value, which is ending oppression. A feminist ethics of health care seeks to foster women's agency where it has previously been restricted by patriarchal patterns and assumptions, and acknowledges that rather than empowering women, the institution of medicine has historically reinforced unequal power relations. Applied to abortion, a feminist ethics of health care identifies the central moral feature of pregnancy as the fact it takes place in women's bodies, and it identifies women and the impact of unwanted pregnancy on their lives as the central element of the moral analysis. It concludes that women, rather than the men in their lives or the government, must control their own reproductive capacity in order to escape oppression.

Critique of Relational, Care, and Feminist Approaches to Abortion Ethics

Taken to their logical extreme, relational theories can lead to odd conclusions. Does a person living alone on an island have no moral standing because no one loves him? If moral status is socially constructed, would a white community's agreement that the one person of color among them isn't a full person make it okay to enslave them? One response would be that a relational approach to abortion ethics rests on a presumption that an embryo or fetus has a lesser moral status than someone who has been born, and therefore analogies involving people do not undermine it.

Care ethics has been criticized as simply reinforcing traditional gender roles. Yes, women are typically the ones doing the work of care, but their investment in this unpaid or low-wage work typically puts them at an economic and political disadvantage. Therefore, without scrutiny of who is caring for whom, a care ethics approach risks simply valorizing the oppression of women.

Sidney Callahan's "pro-life feminism" offers a critique of the traditional feminist position summarized above. She argues that "women can never achieve the fulfillment of feminist goals in a society permissive toward abortion." One line of argument springs from feminism's concern for the oppressed. Women were denied full legal personhood in an earlier era, and now that they have power, it would betray feminist principles for them to turn and revisit that oppression on embryos and fetuses. People have intrinsic moral worth that is distinct from what those in power say they do or don't have, and the same is true of embryos and fetuses—they have an intrinsic moral worth that makes them deserving of care. This intrinsic worth creates a moral obligation for women to nurture this vulnerable creature, which most versions of this argument then transform into a legal obligation. "No prolife feminist would dispute the forceful observations of prochoice feminists about the extreme difficulties that bearing an unwanted child in our society can entail. But the stronger force of the fetal claim presses a woman to accept these burdens," Callahan writes.

A second line of argument springs from feminism's concern for women's well-being. Pro-life feminism disputes that reproductive control contributes to women's equality or happiness. Philosophically, it argues that legal abortion adopts a male model of sex and family and imposes it on women. Practically, Callahan argues that "unless there is an enforced limitation of abortion, which currently confirms the sexual and social status quo, alternatives [that allow women to combine childbearing, education, and careers] will never be developed." She also asserts that women are best served by "the idealized Victorian version of the Christian sexual ethic" (in which sex is embedded within deep emotional bonds and secure long-term commitments, allowing women to enjoy and explore their sexuality across their lifespan in a mutually monogamous relationship in which the man also assumes parental obligations) and argues that abortion bans incentivize this model of male–female relations.

A response to the oppression point is that existing outside another person's body is what those in every other group denied legal personhood in the past have in common, and that refusing to assign personhood to embryos and fetuses because they don't meet this criterion is a logical and reasonable distinction. A response to the equality point is that while the right to abortion certainly doesn't empower women in all respects or solve all social ills, its incomplete effect is no reason to go backward and deprive women of the contributions it does make. Instead, it's a reason to recommit to completing the equality agenda, reminding everyone that support of "choice" means support of childbearing, student and working mothers, and whatever type of sexual relationship a woman wants as well. (This contextualization of reproductive rights as one of many that are needed for women's empowerment is what a reproductive justice agenda provides.) Ironically, the political time and energy consumed by the abortion debate might be one reason we have not yet completed that agenda. Yes, our society still fails to respect the needs of women who want to have children. And pro-life feminism that embraces anti-abortion laws fails to respect the needs of women who *don't* want to have children—ever, at this time, or any more than they already have.

5. MULTI-CRITERION APPROACHES TO ABORTION ETHICS

Single-criterion approaches to abortion ethics, which isolate one thing as the sole relevant factor, are common. We've covered two of them in this chapter—a Human Properties (DNA) approach and a Relational approach—and in the next chapter I discuss the single-criterion approaches of sentience (consciousness as feeling) and cognition (consciousness as thought).

In contrast to single-criterion approaches, multi-criterion* approaches use more than one standard for evaluating the moral status of an entity.

For example, philosopher Bonnie Steinbock (whom I described sharing her abortion story at a conference in Chapter 2) argues that moral status should be ascribed only to beings with interests. In her interests-based approach to reproductive ethics, moral status hinges on what is important to the being itself, rather than what makes that being significant or valuable to others. In order to have interests, beings must have the capacity for conscious awareness and experience. Steinbock considers pain morally significant not for its own sake (pain can be addressed with anesthetic), but because it's arguably the most primitive form of conscious experience. Steinbock says

* Philosophy Fun Fact: The word "criterion" is singular for a standard, so I call these approaches *multi-criterion approaches*. "Criteria" is plural, but because that word is regularly (and incorrectly) used to mean one standard ("that's the third criteria"), calling them "criteria approaches" would be confusing. Philosophers call these approaches "multi-criterial" or "multicriterial," words found in academic literature but not in the dictionary. Therefore, for ease of comprehension, in this section I convert their term to "multi-criterion" throughout.

sentience is the earliest point at which a fetus can be considered as having a life it values, or a life it's possible it enjoys, and therefore a life that could be protected based on its own interests.

At first glance, Steinbock seems to be offering a single-criterion approach. However, while she asserts that "sentience is sufficient for minimal moral status," she also says a sentient fetus can't be given full protection without impermissibly harming the bodily integrity of a being with full moral status, the woman in whom it lives. "For this reason, we cannot simply extend the right to life possessed by all human newborns to sentient fetuses." The combination of these two elements means Steinbock's approach to abortion ethics is ultimately multi-criterion.

Multi-criterion theories that are designed as such are often ambitious attempts to account for the moral status of all living things, or to evaluate the ethics of a wide range of human activity.

One appeal of a multi-criterion approach is it more closely resembles common sense reasoning. People don't usually cling to only one principle, priority, or framework. Instead, we often mix and match multiple values and ways of looking at things, weighing each differently as different situations seem to require.

Using more than one criterion also allows you to temper the extreme conclusions of any single criterion. If rationality is your only criterion for moral standing, it's hard to object to infanticide; adding a relational criterion means a family's love for their not-yet-rational baby can also create moral standing. This is why philosophers Beauchamp and Childress advocate a multi-criterion approach to determining human moral status—because each criterion "falls into implausibility when it loses sight of the merit in competing criteria."

Philosopher Mary Anne Warren agrees that no single principle offers a plausible account of moral status. She offers her own "general account of moral status," a theory that attempts to explain the moral status of all living (and non-living) things, including fetuses. Warren offers seven principles of moral status: the first four concern humans, and the seventh is a unique consideration with particular relevance to the abortion debate. (The fifth and sixth concern plants and animals, which I will overlook for our purposes.)

Warren argues the combination of these four principles determine a particular human's moral status:

1) *The respect for life principle: avoid needless destruction*

Living organisms aren't to be killed or harmed without good reasons that don't violate principles 2 through 7.

2) *The anti-cruelty principle: sentience*

Sentient beings are not to be killed or subjected to pain or suffering, unless there is no other feasible way to further goals that are consistent with principles 3 through 7 and important to human beings.

3) *The agent's rights principle: reasoning*

People who can reason are moral agents, and all moral agents have full and equal basic moral rights, including the rights to life and liberty.

4) *The human rights principle: species membership*

Within the limits of their own capacities and of principle 3, human beings capable of sentience but not of moral agency (such as infants or people with cognitive impairments) have the same moral rights as do moral agents.

Instead of trying to draw an all-or-nothing bright line between "no moral status" and "full moral status," Warren asserts that there are different types of moral status, and they come in varying degrees of strengths. From the highest moral status to the lowest, Warren's categories include:

1. moral agents
2. sentient human beings who are not moral agents
3. sentient nonhuman animals
4. nonsentient living things (plants, ecosystems)

Warren argues that only people in the first category, moral agents (people who can reason), have full moral status based solely upon on their mental and behavioral capacities. People in the second category, sentient humans who are not moral agents (such as infants or people with cognitive impairments), also have full moral status because of relational qualities.

Applying her multi-criterion theory to abortion, Warren concludes that when a fetus has developed sentience, the human rights principle applies, but because it still lives inside a woman, the agent's rights principle that applies to women trumps the second-category status of fetuses.

> Because women are both moral agents and sentient human beings, while first trimester and probably second trimester fetuses are neither, the Agent's Rights principle supports women's right to terminate at any stage before the third trimester. Moreover, although the fetus gains in moral status as it becomes increasingly likely to be capable of sentience, until it has been born it cannot be accorded a fully equal moral status without endangering women's basic rights to life and liberty.

Warren says this "ethical eclecticism" brings moral theory closer to moral common sense, and she places a high priority on common sense as validating moral theory.

Critique of Multi-Criterion Approaches to Abortion Ethics

The complexity of multi-criterion theories is their strength and their weakness. Together the criteria determine the outcome of the analysis, but why those criteria and not others? How can you prove criteria aren't chosen to lead to desired conclusions, and how can you prove one set of criteria is far superior to another? The complexity of multi-criterion approaches might also lead them to lack "inter-rater reliability"—the idea that a valid measure is one that several people can apply independently and still come up with the same results. When criteria come into conflict, which they inevitably do, which prevails? How often people applying the same complex criteria to a nuanced or emotional situation will come to the same conclusion is unclear.

The Transitivity of Respect

Mary Anne Warren's seventh principle for determining moral status is called "the transitivity of respect." This principle doesn't require us to *accept* other people's estimation of moral status. It requires us to *respect* other people enough to give that differing point of view a fair hearing. To the extent it's feasible and morally acceptable, it also requires us to avoid harming entities to which other people ascribe high moral status.

Let's say I'm out hiking, and I come across a rock formation that's a sacred site in a Native American religion. It's not my religion—to me they're just rocks. But to knowingly walk on these rocks would make me a real jerk. I should walk around them, not because I accept the moral status other people assign to these rocks, but out of respect for the people who feel that way. (That's why respect is "transitive" in this principle: I show my respect for people by trying to avoid harming things they treasure.) However, if a bear is nearby and running over those rocks is my best route to safety, it's not feasible or morally required for me to defer to their worldview.

The slogan "Safe, Legal and Rare" has been criticized for suggesting a moral judgment that abortion is bad. "Rare" frames it as a necessary evil we should seek to minimize, stigmatizing and demonizing the women who do have abortions. The transitivity of respect suggests another interpretation of this slogan: "rare" as respect for pluralism.

In a pluralistic society, to say you want abortion to be rare doesn't necessarily mean you think abortion is intrinsically bad. It is an acknowledgment that the existence of abortion causes some of your neighbors anguish, and pluralism requires us to take it easy on our neighbors when we can. We must coexist even though we disagree, so let's reduce friction when possible. This has nothing to do with the legality of abortion; Warren emphasizes that an obligation to respect another's view of embryos or fetuses can never outweigh a woman's moral right to have an abortion under the agent's rights principle. It's about the desirability of reducing unwanted pregnancies. The transitivity of respect would say we should try to make abortion rare not because it is bad, but because it's hard.

The transitivity of respect might also be relevant to the common condemnation of multiple abortions. Say you think the moral status of an embryo is low enough that abortion is morally permissible for any reason at all. Now say a woman is having her second abortion. Do you feel differently about this abortion than you felt about her first? Why? Say it's even her fifth abortion. Surely the moral status of the fifth embryo isn't higher than the first. And the negative effect of delivering an unwanted child is the same for this woman in her fifth pregnancy as it was in the first. So what's the problem?

One reason even some pro-choice people get upset about multiple abortions might be a view that abortion is a permissible way out of trouble, and the fact a woman's decision troubles some of her neighbors is of lesser importance. However, women who keep coming back appear to not be doing their part to avoid either type of trouble. Even if the woman herself thinks embryos have zero moral value, the transitivity of respect would say she ought to respect the fact that some of her neighbors feel otherwise. This view interprets women who have repeat abortions as showing a lack of respect for their neighbors and too heavily taxing our (pluralistic) legal accord. A different analysis would turn the gaze outward, concluding that a woman's repeated need for abortion tells us that her neighbors have failed to respect *her* need for access to things like health care that includes effective contraceptive care, sex education, or personal empowerment within sexual relationships. The fact that in 2014 almost half (45%) of women having an abortion in the U.S. had one previously suggests this is a question worth grappling with.

Turning the transitivity of respect in the other direction encourages kindness to those who favor abortion access. You may not care for abortion, but you cannot deny that some of your neighbors experience it as a critical part of their freedom, and others of your neighbors see its availability as representative of their freedom. Therefore, the transitivity of respect suggests that unless other people's abortions truly threaten your core commitments, respect for these neighbors requires you to respect abortion access.

THE ETHICAL UNDERPINNING OF *ROE V. WADE* AND *CASEY V. PENNSYLVANIA*

The U.S. Supreme Court decisions identifying and affirming the abortion right are driven by constitutional law and legal reasoning, not abortion ethics. However, sometimes legal reasoning coincides with ethical reasoning. Here I simply point out ways in which the law established in *Roe* and *Casey* is consistent with the approaches to abortion ethics reviewed above. This overlap suggests another way to read these decisions—as an expression of the kind of "ethical eclecticism" characteristic of ordinary moral reasoning.

Before viability, the Supreme Court's abortion rulings are consistent with the medical ethics principle of autonomy. *Roe* and *Casey* don't say embryos or fetuses have no moral value. Instead, they rule that the person in whom an embryo or fetus lives, not the government, is the decisionmaker on its moral status. If legislatures pass laws forcing abortion of embryos or fetuses the majority thinks have no moral value, or if they pass laws forcing continued pregnancy for nonviable embryos and fetuses the majority thinks have great moral value, lower courts are obligated to strike these laws. *Roe*'s emphasis on how a woman experiences the burdens of pregnancy is consistent with both the traditional one-person autonomy approach and a two-person analysis. *Casey*'s additional emphasis on how women as a class must have reproductive control to fully participate in society is consistent with an equity of autonomy approach to abortion ethics.

After viability, the Supreme Court's abortion rulings are consistent with a single-intrinsic property (biological) approach to abortion ethics. *Roe* held, and *Casey* affirmed, that a state may take away pregnant women's decisionmaking autonomy after fetuses pass a certain biological point of development (viability) if that state values the potential life of these fetuses more than the needs and desires of the women carrying them. This focus on "potential life" is also consistent with valuing entities in their transitive state because of their potential to be something else. The Court ruled a viable fetus in utero is not a person under the Constitution. Yet because it could become a legal person in the future, a state may assert an interest in protecting it.

Roe required, and *Casey* affirmed, a life-and-health exception to the viability line. In *Doe v. Bolton* (1973), decided the same day as *Roe*, the Court provided a definition of "health" that is consistent with the broad World Health Organization definition that helps drive public health ethics:

> [A physician's] medical judgment may be exercised in the light of all factors—physical, emotional, psychological, familial, and the woman's age—relevant to the wellbeing of the patient. All these factors may relate to health. This allows the attending physician the room he needs to make his best medical judgment. And it is room that operates for the benefit, not the disadvantage, of the pregnant woman.

The life-and-health exception is also consistent with a multi-criterion approach to abortion ethics. States may ban post-viability abortions, except when they're "necessary to preserve the life or health of the mother." The first criterion (the biological status) that the viability standard hinges on has not changed. But a second criterion (the woman's life or health) is added, and it is allowed to change the conclusion. Some people are understandably uneasy about post-viability abortions. But the life-and-health exception is also consistent with a two-person autonomy approach (the ethics of self-defense become relevant here), as well as a relational approach to abortion ethics, because it prioritizes the individual whose absence or impairment would disrupt the larger number of existing relationships.

Finally, the *Roe* Court noted there was no longer a public health rationale for banning abortion. Most state laws criminalizing abortion were first passed in the 19th century, when abortion mortality was high, but by 1973 antiseptic technique and antibiotics reduced the mortality rate of legal abortion to be less than childbirth. The Court's comparison of the death rate of *legal* abortion and childbirth, rather than illegal abortion and childbirth, is consistent with public health ethics, as is its ultimate conclusion, which allows citizens to do what's best for their health.

* * *

You made it! Do you feel more sure? Less sure? More appreciative of other people's thinking? Maybe you found new words for existing certainties, or maybe you changed your mind. Either way, if you're not someone who usually reads philosophy and ethics texts, congratulations.

Bad news. If you answered "yes" on the question of whether abortion is ever ethical, you're not done yet. The next question is: When?

The idea that the moral status of an embryo or fetus increases as it grows is called a gradualist position. Philosopher Maggie Little embraces this school of thought. A process view holds there is a human "substance" that was always there, and only gradually comes into view, like a pile of bricks that eventually becomes a house. "[M]oral status need not be a one-size-fits-all concept: some aspects of status may be present even as other aspects arrive later," Little writes. "At some point, a key common denominator emerges, when the human organism has the fundamental protections of a 'right to life.' Even before this point, though, the life has value; and its status continues to shift after that point is reached." That's why, in Little's view, contraception is preferable to abortion, and early abortion is preferable to later abortion.

But the gradualist intuition doesn't answer the hard questions: does the moral status of an embryo or fetus ever rise higher than the moral status of the woman carrying it? If yes, when do those scales tip, and why?

Chapter 5

Abortion Ethics II

When

The silent story of growth told by the twenty-four museum jars of embryos and fetuses I waddled past when I was pregnant matters to most. As a result, those who answer yes on the Whether question must next consider When.

A biologist once told me his group didn't "know what all the fuss was about" when he invited me to speak about abortion—they knew when life began, so let's see if we couldn't get this whole thing resolved. Our hour together disappointed us both. They left more uncertain than when they came ("Life" as in "person" is a social and moral category that might require more than cellular life? Oh …), and I left kicking myself for having a silly flicker of hope. I knew it was unlikely they had the secret key to ending the abortion debate. But wouldn't it be great if they did?

"Scientism" is the mistake of using science as a moral conclusion. In questions of morality, science is evidence, not argument. Science can't answer our deepest philosophical questions about what it means to be human, social questions about who or what we should care for, or legal questions about who or what has rights. This doesn't mean we should ignore new scientific facts. It means scientific inquiry supplies facts, and ethical inquiry supplies meaning. Embryos and fetuses are liminal creatures in the process of becoming. Science can say when biological attribute X appears. You have to say why X is a moral turning point.

Most When arguments share the same premise: attainment of single-intrinsic property X (a biological feature such as a heartbeat, or lung development, or brain development) is necessary and sufficient for an embryo or fetus to achieve a moral status that trumps the status of the woman carrying it. A strength of single-intrinsic property theories (which for simplicity, I'll refer to as "biological approaches" to the When question) is that they peg abortion limits to something tangible and secular. A claim that embryos or fetuses shouldn't be destroyed after they have X begins with science, not religion.

A weakness of this approach is that it's a jar theory—biological approaches don't mention women. ("Treating women like vessels" is the usual phrasing for approaches that deny or ignore the existence of women, but seeing that exhibit while pregnant has converted them to "jar theories" for me.) As noted in the last chapter, failing to acknowledge that no life exists without the contributions of a woman's body contradicts the biological reality in which these approaches purport to be grounded.

Imagine the reverse: imagine someone proposed an approach to the When question that was exclusively woman-centered. It would revolve around something only the pregnant woman possessed—let's say knowledge. A knowledge approach to abortion ethics might argue that the line distinguishing ethical from unethical abortions (or permissible from impermissible abortions) lies some number of months after a woman learns she's pregnant, or after she learns new information that could reasonably change her decision, such as discovering her husband has abandoned her. In some cases women don't realize they're pregnant or don't get that decision-altering news until very late in pregnancy, so this approach might support some significant number of third-trimester abortions. Doesn't this standard's failure to acknowledge the biological reality of fetal development, in addition to the experiential reality of knowledge, seem inadequate? To some, the failure of jar theories to acknowledge women's experience feels similarly so.

Ignoring the existence of women gives rise to another critique: biological approaches to abortion ethics aren't grounded in a premise of equality. This unspoken premise of inequality is one reason some people find discussion of the moral status of embryos and fetuses offensive or threatening. Suppose a lecturer asks, "Should Asian-American people have equal access to health care?" People will leave in disgust even as he's calling out, "Wait! I was going to prove the answer is yes!" Underneath every question is a claim that this is a question that matters. Beginning from a premise of equality means some questions, like that posed by my imaginary lecturer, just aren't worth asking. From a women's rights perspective, the fetal status question can translate to, "At what point should women lose control of their bodies, such that the state can force them into physical servitude against their will?" Even if the analysis that follows ends in support of abortion rights, some will find the question itself insulting.

That's why talking about the moral value of embryos and fetuses can trigger the intellectual equivalent of an allergic reaction. However, it's hard to avoid those hives. Those who oppose abortion correctly point out that we sometimes curtail liberty for the sake of justice. Bans on child abuse, rape, and slavery protect one person from harm by preventing another person from acting on their personal desires or economic needs. But this reasoning is compelling only if you are convinced of two things: 1) the developing embryo or fetus has interests equivalent to a person who is capable of being abused, raped, or enslaved; and 2) those interests are not outweighed by the fact that—unlike the victim of abuse, rape, and slavery—the fetus lives inside the body of the person who has contrary desires or needs. Discussion of these reasonable analogies requires discussion of the moral status of embryos and fetuses. That's why understanding biological approaches to the When question can be useful to productive exchanges about the ethics of abortion.

The murder of Dr. George Tiller is what first led me to think more deeply about the ethics of When. Dr. Tiller and his colleagues at his Wichita clinic did mostly first- and second-trimester abortions, but they were also among the very few physicians in the country who take care of women in third-trimester cases. They did two types of third-trimester abortions, both of which are legal and rare. The first involves fetuses that can't survive outside the womb because of devastating anomalies. In these cases, there is no legal difference between third-trimester abortion and first-trimester abortion, since both involve fetuses that are not viable. The second type involves viable fetuses when pregnancy threatens the life or health of the woman. The Supreme Court requires states to allow abortion after viability in these circumstances, and Kansas law explicitly allowed abortion after viability when pregnancy would cause "substantial and irreversible impairment of a major bodily function". (K.S.A. 65-6703)

A fellow Kansan named Scott Roeder objected to Dr. Tiller doing what women and couples thought was morally right for them, and what the U.S. Constitution and Kansas law allowed. So one Sunday morning in May 2009, he came to Dr. Tiller's church and, as Dr. Tiller distributed church bulletins and greeted congregants in the doorway, Roeder shot him in the head and killed him.

A few months later I received my first invitation to give an ethics lecture at a national meeting of abortion providers. In addition to immeasurable grief, Dr. Tiller's murder generated a question for his colleagues across the country: Who would take care of these women now? Like patients, health care providers are moral agents who are guided by conscience. This was a meeting of physicians, nurses, and clinic managers who had already answered "yes" to the Whether question—they had all concluded abortion is ethical—but they had different opinions on the When question. Each had a personal line beyond which they were not comfortable providing abortions. Some practiced up to their line, as early or late in pregnancy as it might be. Some faced external obstacles that required them to stop their practice earlier than the line set by their conscience. And some saw pushing themselves past their own personal comfort zone in service of patients in need as an act of conscience. I provided an overview of the ethics of When to help them reflect on whether they should maintain or move their own personal line.

I share a significantly expanded version of that overview in this chapter so you can engage in a similar exercise: What evidence and analyses would lead you to eschew or embrace your legal right to abortion at different points in pregnancy?

Recognizing women, couples, and health care providers as moral thinkers who arrive at a wide range of decisions about abortion, and supporting them as such, is what I think of as a "next generation" conversation in abortion ethics. However, the When question has also become popular with politicians, making discussion of biology, philosophy, medicine, and morality relevant to debates about the limits of government power to ban abortion. Therefore, I note policy examples relevant to each developmental age as well.

A NOTE ON DATES

Pregnancy is often divided into "trimesters," but these three segments aren't equal. According to conception dating (how long the embryo or fetus has been alive), the first trimester ends when a woman has been pregnant 10 weeks. The second trimester encompasses 12 weeks. The third trimester encompasses 16 weeks in a full-term pregnancy.

It's also important to understand the two-week difference between the two systems for calculating gestational age. Because anatomists and obstetricians prefer different ways of dating pregnancy, I use both systems in this section, adding "C" after conception dating and "LMP" after menstrual period dating.

Conception dating (C): This system for dating pregnancy starts counting the day egg and sperm unite. Anatomists and textbooks on human development use conception dating. Their work typically refers to all embryos or fetuses, or to an individual embryo or fetus in the abstract, so their focus is actual age. I use conception dating in this section because single-intrinsic property theories revolve around anatomical milestones in development, and this system of dating identifies when that actually happens.

Last Menstrual Period (LMP) dating: This system for dating pregnancy starts counting from the first day of a woman's last period. Obstetricians working with individual patients use LMP dating. This practice assumes a regular menstrual cycle of 28 days, with ovulation occurring on the 14th day. The expected delivery date is 40 weeks from LMP, which means 38 weeks after conception. (I obsessed over a cutesy week-by-week guide when I was pregnant. The book's chapters describing Week 1 and Week 2 of pregnancy explained ... you're not pregnant yet. Confusing, huh?)

1. Week 0 C/Week 2 LMP: Conception

Policy Example: *Access to emergency contraception*

We considered the DNA/Conception approach to abortion ethics in the last chapter. Here I simply note that it is a biological approach like all the others on this list—it says that egg fertilization is both necessary and sufficient for full moral status. Since the conception line concludes abortion is never ethical, it's traditionally been a Whether argument.

In 2013, the Food and Drug Administration (FDA) approved one of the four brands of emergency contraception (EC) on the market, "Plan B," to be dispensed without a doctor's prescription. The pill is safe, time is of the essence in taking it, and women don't need a doctor's help to "diagnose" whether they've had unprotected sex (consensually or by rape) or a broken condom. However, only eight states currently allow pharmacists to dispense it over the counter.

Does emergency contraception end a pregnancy? Medically, "conception" is not the same as "pregnancy." Conception happens when a sperm fertilizes an egg. After conception, six or more days pass before the fertilized egg travels down the fallopian tube into the uterus, and what has now grown to be a ball of cells called a blastocyst implants into the uterine wall. But over half of all blastocysts fail to implant and simply wash out unnoticed. Therefore, physicians don't call you "pregnant" unless and until implantation has occurred.

However, even if your moral line begins at conception, recent evidence suggests you can take EC. A 2012 article in *The National Catholic Reporter* explains the medical consensus that emergency contraception is not an "abortifacient" (something that causes an abortion). It's a pill that delivers a dose of hormones that delay ovulation. Sperm can survive in a woman's reproductive tract for up to five days, and once an egg is released, the egg can survive up to a day. As a result, intercourse can result in fertilization from five days before ovulation to one day after.

That's why, if taken within 72 hours after intercourse, EC can prevent pregnancy. It does so by preventing an egg from being released while sperm is still alive in a woman's reproductive tract. (The "ella" brand of EC can be taken for all five days.) If an egg has already been fertilized, EC will not prevent that blastocyst from implanting in the uterus, and if it has already been implanted in the uterus, taking EC will not disrupt it.

Yet some still refer to EC as an abortifacient. For example, their belief that EC is an abortifacient was one reason why the family-owned companies that sued in the *Hobby Lobby* case objected to the Affordable Care Act's requirement that insurance plans cover contraception. (They also objected to IUDs on this basis.)

According to the American Congress of Obstetricians and Gynecologists (ACOG), "[o]pponents of EC frequently cite the FDA-approved product label for [products using the hormone in Plan B] which states that 'it may inhibit implantation (by altering the endometrium).' This product label has not been updated since the product was approved in 1999 and does not reflect current research, including recent studies showing that [this hormone] does not cause changes to the endometrium (uterine lining) that would hamper implantation."

It is hard to prove a negative. A conception line that won't allow *any* possibility that EC alters the uterine lining in a way that could prevent implantation of a fertilized egg is extreme and unsustainable as a matter of policy. Of course individuals are free to believe what they like, and to act on those beliefs. Here I simply note that even if there's any way EC could be considered an abortion, it's a legal abortion at the earliest point humanly possible—before a doctor would even say you're pregnant.

So why do 42 states make it harder than necessary for women who want to avoid pregnancy (and potentially also avoid an abortion) to get EC? Can this be construed as abortion opposition? Or is it a state policy of pregnancy as punishment for sex?

2. *Weeks 1–2 C/Weeks 3–4 LMP: Early Embryonic Processes*

Policy Example: *Frozen embryos*

Advances in assisted reproductive technology (ART), such as in vitro fertilization (IVF), have increased scientific knowledge about early embryonic processes. It is now clear that twinning can happen before, but not after, 14 days. Some philosophers focus on individuality as the key to personhood. This science leads them to conclude that an embryo is not a unique entity until the possibility of splitting into two embryos has passed. Religious thinkers focused on ensoulment have cited this line as well. They assert that a soul cannot split in two, and therefore ensoulment cannot happen until fourteen days after conception (4 weeks LMP).

ART has also raised issues that are beyond the scope of this book—such as the moral and legal status of the hundreds of thousands of frozen morulae and blastocysts (commonly referred to as embryos, although they're under a week old) that couples have made, then left behind in frozen storage in U.S. fertility clinics. Here I simply note that courts usually give couples who disagree (for example, after divorce) equal say on what shall become of embryos that exist outside a woman's body. If the man doesn't want to procreate, the woman can't use them, and vice versa.

According to Professor Steinbock's interest-based approach (described in Chapter 4), abortion doesn't wrong embryos or preconscious fetuses because they have no stake in what happens to them. However, Steinbock argues that entities without moral *status* (because they do not have interests) can still have what she calls moral *standing*, which is a claim on our moral attention. Steinbock argues that an embryo is a potential person that serves as a symbol of human life, and this potential and symbolic value means it deserves more respect than human cells lacking these qualities. Therefore, she argues, while embryos don't have a moral status that warrants "Golden Rule" treatment in which we consider their interests (because they have none), and therefore they may be used for stem cell research, their moral standing means they deserve a respect that prohibits them from being put to frivolous or trivial uses in a laboratory.

3. *Week 4 C/Week 6 LMP: Heartbeat*

Policy Example: *North Dakota banned abortion after a fetal heartbeat is detected. In 2013 a federal appellate court ruled the ban was unconstitutional because it violates all the Supreme Court precedents setting the line at viability, and the U.S. Supreme Court declined to review the decision. In 2016 Ohio passed a ban on abortion after a heartbeat can be detected, and several other state legislatures considered one, but none became law.*

Cultural Example: *"Abortion Stops a Beating Heart" billboards.*

Abortion Experience: *32% of U.S. abortions occur before 6 weeks LMP, 66% before 8 weeks LMP.*

The cardiovascular system is the first organ system to function. The heart begins as a single tube that starts contracting 3 weeks after conception (22 days), which is 5 weeks LMP. That's referred to as "seeing" a heartbeat. In the typical doctor's office the contractions of the heart tube can be seen with vaginal ultrasound around 6 weeks LMP.

"Heartbeat" usually connotes something we can *hear*. The "lub-dub" sound of a heartbeat is caused by the closing of the heart valves, so a heartbeat can't be heard before the chambers are partitioned and the valves are complete. The heart partitions into chambers over the course of approximately a month (Weeks 4–8 after conception/Weeks 6–10 LMP). So, anatomically, the earliest possible time to hear a heartbeat is after about 9 weeks LMP. The ultrasound instrument used in the typical obstetrician's office, a hand-held Doppler, usually doesn't pick up the sound of a heartbeat until 10–12 weeks LMP.

The ethical argument in favor of a heartbeat line might rely on symmetry with the old heart-lung standard for declaring death: a person is dead after his or her heart stops beating. Therefore an embryo with a heartbeat is "alive."

The problem with this logic is that an embryo that's been around for 4 weeks has been "alive" since conception, so that is not a new status in and of itself. Regardless, "alive" is not synonymous with "person" (many things are alive), and "person" is not the opposite of "dead" (an adult whose heart has stopped beating remains a person; she is now a dead person). So from here a second argument must be made explaining why the version of "alive" that includes a heartbeat is a morally definitive turning point marking a new moral status equal to persons outside the womb.

4. *Week 9 C/Week 11 LMP: The shift from embryo to fetus*

Policy Example: *The regulation of medication abortion ("the abortion pill").*

Cultural Example: *Size and looks are often used rhetorically in abortion discussion, debate, and protests.*

Abortion Experience: *80% of abortions take place before Week 11 LMP.*

An embryo becomes a fetus at the end of the 8th week after conception. This change in terminology marks a large turning point in development: Day 1 of Week 9 (C)/Week 11 (LMP) is when every organ system's basic structure is in place. (This explains why the risk of miscarriage declines significantly as pregnancy advances.)

Significant external changes are completed in the transition from embryo to fetus as well. Before Week 11 begins it's hard to tell what species this creature belongs to; in Week 11 it looks human. Eyes, ears, and nose are visible on a face, the embryonic tail has disappeared, and limbs with fingers and toes are complete. Yet when it's first called a fetus, it's just over one inch—its "crown to rump" length (the standard measurement) is 30 millimeters.

The week an embryo becomes a fetus is rarely mentioned in ethics or law, but I mention it here as a proxy for appearance. Looks matter in the public abortion conversation. People opposing abortion rights often show magnified pictures of fetuses with recognizably human faces, and people supporting abortion rights often point out how small an embryo is. They're making a similar, usually implicit, claim—that after fetuses look like "one of us," they should be protected, and before they reach a size that makes them recognizable as "one of us," they need not be protected. And pro-fetal rights advocates commonly use the word "fetus" to encompass every stage of pregnancy, perhaps because its connotation of "something with a face" inspires more sympathy than "embryo."

Philosophically, the looks argument is weak. Yet Dr. Sarah McNeil, who teaches family medicine residents in San Francisco how to do abortions, told me the developmental difference between embryos and fetuses matters to her trainees. In her experience, the difference between looking at unidentifiable tissue and seeing recognizable fetal body parts "gives most residents pause." Their reaction confirms an obvious statement: looks are powerful. Even if you think the development of qualities like breathing or cognition is more morally significant than appearance, on a gut level, "that looks like a baby" goes a long way. But not all the way. "For those [residents] committed to providing services," Dr. McNeil continued, "they think about seeing fetal parts, ponder life and death and their role in all of this, and decide that seeing fetal parts would not stop them." When I first mentioned the "looks" line in a presentation I thought I was just talking about political rhetoric. Dr. McNeil's comment reminded me of something you'd think I'd know by now: that doctors are people too.

A second reason I mention this line is that it corresponds perfectly with the FDA's recent extension allowing Mifeprex to be used through the 10th week of pregnancy. Mifeprex is called RU-486 in Europe and "the abortion pill" in the United States. The abortion pill essentially causes a first-trimester miscarriage. Some patients prefer it because they can experience those effects at home, and they can do so at a time that works for them (such as after their children are asleep instead of office hours). In 2014, medication abortions accounted for 31% of all nonhospital abortions and 45% of all abortions before 9 weeks LMP.

However, for the 16 years that the abortion pill has been legal in the United States, it's been burdened by what's called a "REMS"—special restrictions imposed by the FDA that, in this case, do not improve safety. Your doctor can't write a prescription for Mifeprex for you to fill at the pharmacy like almost every other drug. Instead, doctors must give you the pill in his or her office. In order to have Mifeprex in their office, your doctor must become "certified," which means they must put their name on a national list of "certified abortion providers," and endure the expense and inconvenience of stocking a drug in their offices.

These regulations reduce the potential benefits of the abortion pill by making it harder to get. Understandably, some physicians who would be willing to write a normal prescription for the abortion pill to their patients with unwanted first-trimester pregnancies are not willing to jump through these extra hoops. The result of these regulations is that instead of providing integrated care, these physicians have to refer their patients out to abortion clinics. Requiring a second appointment at a clinic which might be hours away from patients' homes unnecessarily delays abortion and burdens patients.

Factors like these led the authors of a recent article in *The New England Journal of Medicine* to call for this special regulation of Mifeprex to be lifted.

5. *Weeks 14–16 C/Weeks 16–18 LMP: "Quickening"*

Policy Example: *For centuries in Europe, and later in the United States, abortion was not a crime before the woman first felt the fetus move, which was called "quickening." This often happens between 16 and 18 weeks LMP, but variations in physical factors can push it as late as 22 or 24 weeks for some women.*

Abortion Experience: *95% of U.S. abortions happen before Week 16 LMP.*

Quickening was the dominant biological approach to the When question for centuries. I'm struck by the fact that 95% of women who have abortions in the United States do so before the possibility of quickening—before Week 16—even though legally they have approximately another two months before viability to do it.

However, it wouldn't be accurate to say the way 95% of American women vote with their feet represents collective moral reasoning that abortion before quickening is better than after. Psychologically, a pregnant woman who knows she doesn't want to have a baby might want closure as soon as possible. Physically, she has no incentive to continue enduring pregnancy symptoms like nausea and exhaustion. And socially, she has a strong incentive to terminate before her pregnancy shows. (First pregnancies typically start showing between 18 and 24 weeks, but subsequent pregnancies can show as early as 14 to 16 weeks.) Abortion becomes more expensive and the difficulty of finding a provider increases as pregnancy progresses, so structural barriers might also drive women to take action earlier.

I'm not aware of any contemporary proponents of fetal movement as an ethically determinative turning point, and through sonography we now know fetal movement happens before a fetus is big enough for a woman to feel it. I mention it here simply to point out that quickening is the only developmental line on this list besides delivery that pregnant women know from their own physical experience. Perhaps that's why several abortion providers have told me that in their experience, it's hard for women to ask for abortion after they feel movement, and when they do, it's usually because something is seriously wrong with the woman or the fetus.

6. *Week 22 C/Week 24 LMP: Viability*

> ***Policy Example:*** Roe v. Wade *(1973): "With respect to the State's important and legitimate interest in potential life, the 'compelling' point is at viability. This is so because the fetus then presumably has the capability of meaningful life outside the mother's womb. State regulation protective of fetal life after viability thus has both logical and biological justifications."*

In *Roe* the Supreme Court chose lung development as the point after which states can ban abortion if that's the policy they want.

In the uterus, an embryo or fetus gets oxygen from the pregnant woman. Her lungs deliver oxygen to her blood, and that oxygen passes to its blood through the placenta. In an otherwise healthy fetus, viability is the point at which its lungs are developed enough that they could transfer oxygen into its own blood, either independently or with the support of a ventilator, if the umbilical cord were to be cut.

"Viable" doesn't mean "100% chance of survival." *Roe* says viability occurs when a fetus is "potentially able to live outside the mother's womb. . . ." When *Casey* affirmed the viability standard in 1992, it described viability as a "realistic possibility of maintaining and nourishing a life outside the womb."

What odds capture "potentially able," and what's a "realistic possibility"? The Supreme Court left that to us. Current medical practice puts viability at roughly 24 weeks, so "elective" abortions typically stop at 23 weeks and 6 days LMP. Of neonates delivered prematurely in Week 24, 62% survived to discharge, according to a large study of academic medical centers across the country between 2008 and 2012.*

The *Roe* viability standard isn't just brute survival, it includes a quality-of-life assessment—a viable fetus is one capable of "meaningful life." But *Roe* also leaves us to define "meaningful," and what the odds of attaining that meaningful state must be in order to be called viable. In the study mentioned above, 89% of the survivors in Week 24 had what the researchers classified as a "major morbidity," which means a major health problem.**

Many doctors and institutions use 24 weeks as a proxy for viability, which means current medical practice interprets "a realistic possibility of a meaningful life" to mean an approximately 62% chance of survival, and an 11% chance of surviving without a major morbidity, if taken out of the womb. However, the Supreme Court has confirmed that states cannot reduce the concept of viability to a number of weeks specified in a statute (*Colautti v. Franklin*, 1979), and viability is still an assessment the law leaves to individual physicians and patients. That's one reason you hear experts say, "viability, which is *around* 24 weeks." Another reason is that a fetus with devastating health problems might not be "viable" at any gestational age, meaning that if that nonviable fetus was delivered prematurely at 32

* For comparison, the survival rates for the surrounding weeks were as follows: 7% at 22 weeks LMP; 32% at 23 weeks; 77% at 25 weeks. The increasing survival odds are linked to the development of a crucial bit of anatomy called alveoli. Alveoli are the tiny saclike structures that transfer oxygen from the lungs to the blood. If they haven't developed yet, gas exchange is impossible, and delivering air through a ventilator won't save that baby.

** The major morbidity rates for the surrounding weeks were as follows: 100% at 22 weeks; 95% at 23 weeks; 78% at 25 weeks LMP. There isn't a standard definition of what conditions are "major morbidities." In this study, these ranged from conditions that could lead to death after discharge, problems that could require significant home health care needs for life (such as a bad brain bleed), problems that wouldn't stop typical development if they were overcome (such as a terrible infection), and disabilities such as blindness that some would call "major" and others would call "minor."

weeks, resuscitation would not be offered. Finally, today neonatologists look at a combination of factors when making an individualized assessment. (For example, a big singleton girl at 23 weeks has a better chance of survival than a small twin boy at 25 weeks.)

According to the Supreme Court, a fetus is not a "person" as the word is used in the Constitution. Yet in the last four months of pregnancy, the Court allows states to assert an interest in fetal life that trumps a woman's interest in bodily integrity. According to *Casey*, that's because at this point of lung development, "the independent existence of the second life can, in reason and all fairness, be the object of state protection that now overrides the rights of the woman."

There's a rarely recognized disjuncture between the moral justification of the lung line and the way it actually works in practice. The Supreme Court decided that the point at which a fetus no longer needs a woman's body to survive is when the state can force that woman to remain pregnant. I call this the viability paradox.

Once a fetus can survive *outside* a woman's body, *Roe* and *Casey* conclude she can be compelled by law to keep it *inside* her body for the remaining four months of pregnancy. What led the Court to decide this? According to *Roe*:

> The pregnant woman cannot be isolated in her privacy. She carries an embryo and, later, a fetus … it is reasonable and appropriate for a State to decide that at some point in time another interest … that of potential human life, becomes significantly involved. The woman's privacy is no longer sole and any right of privacy she possesses must be measured accordingly.

This passage raises two key questions the Court has never answered. If embryos and fetuses are never "persons" under the Constitution while they are in a woman's uterus, why are pregnant women no longer alone? From a constitutional perspective, exactly who (or what) else is there rendering a pregnant woman no longer "sole," no longer "isolated"? The *Roe* Court does not raise or address these questions. It just states that the right of personal privacy is "not unqualified" and the abortion right is not "absolute," without offering any more argument for its conclusion.

Many assume that what the Court balanced against women's right to privacy is fetal rights, but it was not. Instead, the Court identified a "state interest" in "potential human life." This raises the second key question: What justifies the government's interest in something inside a woman's body that is not a "person" under the Constitution? A governmental interest in creating more taxpayers? More soldiers? The *Roe* Court never explains why exactly the state has an interest in prenatal life sufficient to override its citizens' interest in bodily integrity and family formation after viability. An argument from pluralism on the When question might say abortion decisions should be left to the consciences of women, families, and their physicians throughout pregnancy.

The *Roe* Court's decision that a fetus isn't a legal "person" until birth, yet states can force women to continue pregnancies against their will for the last four months of pregnancy, is a significant intrusion on bodily privacy and liberty that's rarely analyzed. In this sense, *Roe* itself is a major compromise.

At the end of this chapter I argue there are good reasons for keeping the viability standard. However, the burden on women who are legally compelled to carry unwanted pregnancies after viability is underappreciated.

7. *Week 22 C/Week 24 LMP or later: Sentience (the capacity to feel pain)*

Policy Example: *As of June 2017, eighteen states banned abortion based on their assertion of when a fetus can feel pain. Mississippi asserts this happens at 18 weeks (C)/20 weeks (LMP); the*

> *others assert it happens at 20 weeks (C)/22 weeks (LMP). In two other states, pain bans were found unconstitutional by a federal appellate court because they violate "a long line of invariant Supreme Court precedents" setting the line at viability. In 2013, the U.S. Supreme Court declined to review the decision on Arizona's pain ban, and in 2015, Idaho did not appeal its appellate court loss on its pain ban to the Supreme Court.*

There are two places one could locate the capacity to feel pain in this list of single-intrinsic-property theories. Scientists and physicians put it after viability, so that's where I've put it on this list. Some legislators put it before viability. But we can analyze the ethical significance of this developmental turning point without debating which week it occurs.

"Sentience" is the capacity to experience pain and pleasure. Researchers haven't pinpointed exactly what week that capacity emerges, but the scientific consensus is that whatever week it occurs, it cannot be earlier than 26 weeks, and it more likely occurs much later in the third trimester.

A 2005 review of the literature published in *JAMA* concluded that "the capacity for functional pain perception in preterm neonates probably does not exist before 29 or 30 weeks. . . . Evidence regarding the capacity for fetal pain is limited but indicates that fetal perception of pain is unlikely before the third trimester."

In 2010, the Royal College of Obstetricians and Gynecologists (the British equivalent of ACOG) reviewed the evidence and came to a similar conclusion. It added that

> there is increasing evidence that the fetus never experiences a state of true wakefulness *in utero* and is kept, by the presence of its chemical environment, in a continuous sleep-like unconsciousness or sedation. This state can suppress higher cortical activation in the presence of intrusive external stimuli. This observation highlights the important differences between fetal

> and neonatal life and the difficulties of extrapolating from observations made in newborn preterm infants to the fetus. ... [Therefore], there appeared to be no clear benefit in considering the need for fetal analgesia prior to termination of pregnancy, even after 24 weeks, in cases of fetal abnormality.

In 2013, ACOG issued its statement. It describes "pain" as an emotional and psychological experience that requires conscious recognition of a noxious stimulus. A developing human needs two things to feel pain. First is the physiological capacity to feel. The connections that send nerve signals to the brain, and the brain structures that process those signals, are not in place until at least 24 weeks. These structures are necessary, but not sufficient, for sentience. The second thing needed to feel pain is the "neural circuitry" to distinguish painful touch from any touch, a capacity that doesn't develop until late in the third trimester, ACOG explained.

If legislators want to substitute "pain" as we usually think of it for viability, that new line would allow elective abortion into the third trimester. If they want to use "pain" to mean development of some "physical structures" necessary for experiencing it (the language of some of the 20-week pain bans) even though those structures are not sufficient, that change would keep the line at about the same point as the current viability line (around 24 weeks) under a different rationale.

Philosopher Peter Singer argues abortion is morally neutral before fetuses can feel pain. He doesn't argue abortion is impermissible after the capacity to feel pain develops, but Singer uses pain as a morally defining feature to expand the list of creatures to which we owe moral obligations to include both animals and human. Singer considers elements like rationality, self-conscious awareness, autonomy, pleasure and pain as the morally relevant criteria for personhood. Therefore, he concludes that the wrongness of causing pain or of killing depends on the degree of development, not the species to which a creature belongs.

8. *Weeks 25–32 C/Weeks 27–34 LMP: Organized cortical activity*

> ***Policy Example:*** Roe *and* Casey *require states to allow post-viability abortions if pregnancy threatens a pregnant woman's life or health.* Roe *and* Casey *permit, but do not require, states to ban other abortions after viability. As of April 2017, seven states do not ban other post-viability abortions.*

"Brain death" marks the end of a person's life. I think of this biological approach to the When question as proposing a bookend to that—"brain birth."

Philosopher David Boonin argues that fetuses acquire a moral status that confers a "right to life" when their brains can produce brain waves like you and I have. Organized cortical activity is the developmental point at which fetuses move from the capacity to feel (sentience) to the capacity to think (cognition). He calls this "the cortical criterion" for short.

Random electrical activity begins earlier in development, but somewhere in the range of 25–32 weeks after conception, a fetus's brain begins to produce the continuous electroencephalograph (EEG) waves you see when a large number of synapses have formed. (Normal EEG that is at least somewhat like that of an adult doesn't appear until shortly after birth.)

What's significant about the shift from random (also called "burst") activity to organized cortical activity? Boonin argues that desires are what's necessary to trigger a moral status justifying a "right to life." Conscious experience must be present for a being to have desires, and conscious experience can't possibly happen until the brain develops organized cortical activity.

How can a fetus have desires? Boonin's focus is a type of deep, unconscious desire. What you're consciously thinking right now (like "I wish this chapter was shorter") is called an occurrent desire.

The desires you have at an unconscious level (like "I'd like to live past tomorrow") are called dispositional desires. You aren't "thinking" your dispositional desires, but you still have them.

Take an adult who's temporarily unconscious. She has no occurrent (conscious) desire to live. But, Boonin says, we treat her in response to her underlying dispositional desire to live—a desire we all have once we have the brain anatomy to generate it. For Boonin, a fetus is "one of us" after organized cortical activity, because at that point it's capable of having the underlying dispositional desire for continued survival we all have.

I applied the term "brain birth" to help us think about Boonin's argument, but it's important to note what he's describing is not perfectly symmetrical to brain death. Brain death is a total, and often abrupt, loss of all brain function ("irreversible cessation of all functions of the entire brain, including the brain stem"), while what I'm calling "brain birth" is an already living brain's shift toward organized activity. "Brain birth" is understood through EEG; brain death is diagnosed by physical examination, and EEG is only an ancillary, optional test in that process.

However, Boonin's argument does not turn on this symmetry (or lack thereof). His argument turns on dispositional desires, which both a young fetus and a brain-dead adult lack the neurological ability to generate.

9. *Weeks 38–40 C/Weeks 40–42 LMP: Delivery*

Birth results in actual separation from a woman's body—as opposed to theoretical or potential separation—and the end of dependency on another's body. Newborns still depend on physical care to survive, but now that care can be provided by others if needed. Birth also involves a physiological change. Before birth, blood bypasses a fetus's nonfunctioning lungs in two temporary "shunts." However, the fetal circulatory system is designed to be able to convert to the adult pattern with the first breath. So the first breath marks a "system switch" from dependent to independent, which one could argue marks a change in moral status.

Mary Anne Warren, the philosopher who offered the multi-criterion approach discussed earlier, asserts that birth is the appropriate point to fully enforce the human rights principle as it applies to sentient human beings. This position addresses the concern of the "viability paradox" (explained above) because it's based on where the baby actually lives, not where it theoretically could live.

A "MORAL COHERENCE" DEFENSE OF VIABILITY

Earlier I critiqued the viability line for failing to match its moral claim (this is when fetuses could live outside women's bodies) with its experiential outcome (therefore it's when women are required to keep fetuses inside their bodies). Legally, one could argue that because *Roe* decided a fetus is not a "person" within the meaning of the Constitution, abortion decisions should be left to conscience throughout pregnancy.

So why haven't those who support abortion's legality tried to push *Roe*'s viability line forward with the same energy that those who oppose abortion's legality have tried to roll it back?

Perhaps it's because post-viability abortions challenge what philosophers call "coherence of attitudes." In ethics it's called casuistry, in law it's called precedent, in life it's called fairness—the desire to see like cases treated alike.

In a period neonatologists call "the gray zone," parents get to decide how to respond to premature delivery: whether to try to resuscitate the neonate, or whether to allow it to die (as it inevitably will without aggressive resuscitation and continuing interventions) with comfort care to make that death peaceful. There is some variation in practice, but when the neonate has no health problems in addition to prematurity, this zone is generally considered to be from about 22 weeks to 25 weeks. Before 22 weeks there's no point in even trying resuscitation; at 25 weeks most doctors and hospitals say the odds of success are high enough that they don't allow parents to say no. (This is not standardized—some hospitals draw this line at 26 weeks.)*

This means that an obstetrician might do an abortion at 23 weeks and 6 days LMP in one room of a hospital, then run to another to do a delivery at the exact same age for a neonate parents want aggressively resuscitated.

Location is a key difference in these cases: premature labor has expelled the fetus in the second case from the woman's body, shifting its source of life support from woman to world, and shifting its legal and social category from fetus to baby. Another key difference is the women's desires: in the first case the patient doesn't want to become a mother, and in the second case she does. For several hospital-based obstetricians I know who have been in this situation, together those differences are enough.

Beyond about 24 weeks, that dissonance would be hard to sustain. I suspect the number of fetuses that leave the womb at 25 weeks and still survive to be healthy children makes abortion after 25 weeks feel different. It's not that the capacity for independent breathing is what makes you "one of us." It's that we've seen a significant number of neonates that can breathe *become* one of us. As a result, culturally, socially, psychologically, and experientially, a later cut-off for abortions done for reasons other than health might feel incoherent.

* Interestingly, physicians and hospitals allow parents to decline potentially life-saving interventions for premature infants that have odds of success higher than they would be allowed to decline for older children. Perhaps this is a variation on the "looks" argument discussed above—at 25 weeks, the average neonate weighs about 1.5 pounds. It can be argued that the wider latitude for parental decisionmaking at this stage is discrimination, or it's a collective cultural assessment that the moral status of babies that leave the womb early in the third trimester is lower than older babies and children.

Perhaps this is what Justice O'Connor was getting at when in *Casey* she wrote for the majority that "there is no line other than viability which is more workable."

The "brain birth" standard appeals to me intellectually, but the psychological dissonance that standard might cause for physicians who both deliver babies and do abortions might be overwhelming. Neonatologists have feelings around this too—for example, one pro-choice neonatologist told me the idea of aborting a healthy 26-week fetus makes her sad not because she sees some survive, but because she sees so many babies die whose parents are desperate for them to live. It would be fair to say these conflicts are for these doctors to work out; they can continue or alter their medical practice as they like. But I see the potential response of obstetricians and neonatologists as foreshadowing a broader cultural dissonance that would be hard to sustain.

Another way in which the viability standard is morally coherent is that it's the only biological approach reviewed in this chapter that is not a jar theory. Viability acknowledges and addresses the fact that embryos and fetuses depend on a woman's body for their survival. Before viability they die without her. The viability standard makes the potential for change in that *relationship* pivotal. The viability paradox (perhaps summarized by *Casey* calling a viable fetus living inside a woman's body "independent life") diminishes this relational strength of the lung line. But viability is the only biological line with any relational aspect at all.

The capacity to feel pain is less compelling than viability. It's morally incoherent in two ways. Defining the capacity to feel pain as what marks a creature sufficiently "one of us" that it can't be killed suggests there's no such thing as "humane" killing of animals that also feel pain—so shall eating meat be made illegal too? The second incoherence is the same as the brain birth standard. Honest application of the best science available means replacing viability with capacity to feel pain would extend the constitutional right to abortion beyond *Roe*'s approximately 24 weeks LMP to 26 weeks or later.*

Moral coherence may explain why it made intuitive sense to the majority of Justices in *Roe* and *Casey* to identify viability as the point after which states may ban abortion (unless the pregnancy threatens the life or health of the woman) with little supporting argument. And the viability paradox explains why the few states that have not exercised their option of banning abortion after viability, and have instead left abortion decisions to the consciences of patients and doctors throughout pregnancy, have also made a defensible choice.

WHETHER, WHEN . . . AND WHY?

A patient's pregnancy was days from viability, and her physicians were afraid practical obstacles might prevent them from performing her abortion before she crossed the line. Hospital staff who usually opposed abortion, especially in the second trimester, seemed unconcerned about the viability threshold. "Just do it!" they urged the surprised physicians.

Why? Because the patient was 10 years old. *Ten.* A family member had gotten her pregnant. And it wasn't until Week 23 that a relative finally noticed something different about this little girl's body. For some members of the hospital staff, the extraordinary reasons for this patient's abortion outweighed the tremendous moral value they assigned to viability.**

* If future science proved fetuses could feel pain before viability, that would be a winning argument for using fetal anesthesia during abortion. But to my mind, the moral arguments in favor of viability would remain superior.

** The physicians were firm—at their hospital they never go beyond the viability line, and if they had not been able to see this patient before 23 weeks and 6 days LMP, they would

Did you notice that in all the pages you've just plowed through, not one of the approaches to abortion ethics reviewed in Chapters 4 and 5 takes into account the *reason* a woman wants an abortion? (The only one that arguably does that is the autonomy approach—but it does so indirectly by deferring to whatever reason the decisionmaker decides is sufficient.)

Reasons are irrelevant to the law. (Except after viability, when the reason of a health threat becomes relevant.) Yet in private conversation, reasons are central to women and couples considering abortion, and to people judging others' abortion decisions.

Considering reasons along with embryonic or fetal moral status could be called a multi-criterion ethics approach to abortion. In everyday moral reasoning, women considering abortion weigh factors all patients weigh: their values, their circumstances, their needs, the desires of others they love, and their hopes for the future.

Reasons are also inextricably bound with your assessment of the moral status of embryos and fetuses. If you rank that moral status highly, only extraordinary reasons will outweigh it for you. If you rank it lowly, a wide range of ordinary reasons will justify abortion for you. And because for most people moral status changes over time, reasons sufficient for a woman to feel okay about ending her pregnancy at Week 2 or 3 might seem insufficient to her at Week 23.

not have performed an abortion. (As explained above, states can't substitute a number for the concept of viability, but hospitals can make policies for themselves.) After viability this patient would qualify for a legal abortion under the life-and-health exception (which includes consideration of mental health, as well as age), but the rules of every hospital in this large liberal city meant that even post-viability abortions that are legal couldn't be done there. Instead, this little girl would have had to fly to one of the few facilities in the country that do third-trimester procedures. (This case reminded me of a similar case described at a memorial service for Dr. Tiller, the Kansas physician who was murdered in 2009. A patient of a similar age and circumstance had to fly to his clinic for an abortion. Anticipating that this traumatized child would be terrified to be away from home among medical personnel she'd never met before, Dr. Tiller had pink t-shirts made that the entire clinic staff wore the day she arrived, all of which said "Friend of [name].") In the end, the patient described above did not have to fly—they were able to perform the abortion just before viability.

Yet regular people barely talk about abortion, and when they do, they don't talk like philosophers. That means you have to make the connection between reasons, and what those reasons tell you about what moral status the woman or couple assign to embryos or fetuses.

The problem with discussion of "good" and "bad" reasons for abortion is that when people disagree about the moral status of embryos and fetuses, they assess reasons differently too. Seventy-four percent of women having abortions say having a baby would interfere with work, school, or their ability to care for dependents. To say those reasons aren't "good enough" is to impose a singular assessment of the moral value of embryos and fetuses on these women's consciences and bodies.

Writer Katha Pollitt argues that the idea women should carry every zygote they create shows "disregard for the seriousness of motherhood." Pollitt is right that choosing to have a child is a morally significant decision, and parenting is a serious moral commitment. That's why I agree with those who want to reclaim the moral seriousness of "I don't want to be a parent" as a reason for abortion.

However, notice that Pollitt's analysis doesn't challenge the high moral status implicitly granted to that zygote. Instead, it matches it by arguing (by analogy to motherhood) that "I don't want to be a parent" is a reason that weighs even more. That's fine. All I'm saying is that in the United States, you're also allowed to think an embryo does not have any moral significance, just as your neighbor is free to think it is the moral equivalent of a child.

"Pro-choice" doesn't mean you don't have opinions about other people's choices, or that you can't think a woman is wrong about moral status. To be "pro-choice" is to recognize that your neighbor is a moral thinker too. In a pluralistic society, she's allowed to disagree with your assessment, and you must have reciprocal respect for each other's conclusions.

However, in this book I've analyzed other people's situations, and perhaps you followed suit. So which is it—do we get to judge other people's reasons or not?

I invite you to consider "cases" the way we do in ethics. Humans analyze other people's situations to make sense of the world, to get a grasp on how things are and how they could or should be. Considering another person's actions allows us to contemplate what we might do in comparable circumstances. When you approve or disapprove of the behavior of others, you learn something about yourself. Thinking "I don't approve of that person's action" teaches you that were you to find yourself in a parallel situation, that action wouldn't be right for you.

Perhaps that's why the phrase "don't judge me" has always struck me as odd. Blame my legal training, but "judgment" isn't necessarily a bad word to me. ("Cute haircut!" is also a judgment, but people rarely object when judgment is positive—that's called a compliment.) Done well, "judgment" is a reasoned analysis and fair-minded conclusion. Given that, perhaps "don't judge me" (or "don't judge people") could be understood as a rejection of this activity done poorly: "Don't judge me unfairly—withhold your judgment until you understand all the facts. Don't judge me without empathy—understand that I and my life are different from you and yours, and I am the only one who can and will live mine."

It's also helpful to remember that a judge is only empowered to assess the situations of parties that ask for his or her intervention. (Only one party asks; the other might be quite unhappy to have been dragged there.) This suggests that judgment of people who don't put their situations in the public eye, or people who don't disclose them to you personally and seek your opinion, is out of your jurisdiction.

When you disagree with someone's reasons for abortion, understand that what's really happening is you two disagreeing on the moral status of embryos or fetuses. Moving from judgment of reasons to disagreement on moral status can help us productively discuss our true conflict. And even if that discussion doesn't change either person's mind, your analysis might help clarify your own values. I've told abortion stories that I hope inspire you to think about other people's choices, but not so you can "sit in judgment of them." I offer them to help you judge what's right and wrong for yourself.

Earlier I noted that American women have 2.8 million unintended pregnancies a year, and 42% of them end in abortion. This book focuses on the prevalence of abortion because I think these little known numbers are significant. However, we shouldn't forget the other side of that statistic, which is the 58% of women with unintended pregnancies who proceed to delivery (such as Betty, mentioned in Chapter 3). This group is also making choices based on their values, circumstances, and vision of their future, yet these women are oddly invisible in our examination of abortion. Remembering them reminds us of the obvious—that Americans have different beliefs, and take different actions. I think all of them deserve our respect.

Chapter 6

Abortion Politics

Trojan Horses, Russian Dolls, and Realpolitik

In 2013 Texas passed a new law: abortion clinics had to meet the same construction standards as ambulatory surgical centers (ASCs), and physicians couldn't perform abortions unless they had admitting privileges to a hospital within 30 miles of the clinic. Sounds reasonable enough, right?

The hitch is these "improvements" in abortion care wouldn't make an already safe procedure any safer. So why were they added? The Texas Legislature said it was to protect women's health. However, those who follow these things—both opponents and supporters of abortion rights—knew that wasn't true. Oddly, one question in *Whole Woman's Health v. Hellerstedt* (2016) was whether the U.S. Supreme Court was allowed to see and say the facts.

American abortion politics has a Trojan Horse problem: most abortion laws crafted to appear as if they protect patients are really meant to protect embryos and fetuses. It also has a Russian Doll problem: arguments about the moral value of embryos and fetuses sometimes contain hidden agendas on other important social issues. The misdirection of Trojan Horses and Russian Dolls wastes ordinary citizens' time and energy on false questions and keeps American abortion politics stuck in the mud. Recognizing this defect in our public abortion conversation would help us save our energy for the honest, hard questions that might move us forward. What are those questions? That's an issue of Realpolitik I address at the end.

But first: Why would a bioethics book include a chapter on politics? Because understanding where power lies and how it's deployed is part of our job. When that analysis concerns governmental action, bioethicists are called to be "political" in the classic sense—concerned with policymaking.

I. TROJAN HORSES

In Texas, those in the know understood that the 2013 statute was a Trojan Horse abortion law because there was no evidence the new construction standards, such as requiring patients swallowing the abortion pill to be standing in a multimillion-dollar operating room when they do it, would improve abortion's already enviable safety record. Your odds of dying from a colonoscopy are ten times higher than dying from an abortion. But Texas doesn't require colonoscopy to be performed in an ASC, and the new regulations didn't apply to other medical specialties or procedures in Texas with safety records comparable to abortion, just abortion clinics. Requiring admitting privileges wouldn't improve safety either. Admitting privileges are a formal arrangement that typically allow a doctor to admit a patient to a hospital under his or her name and to treat that patient while he or she is in the hospital. However, all hospitals are required to treat all patients when there's an emergency, and they have the specialized medical staff to do so. (It's also the case that when the rare complication of an abortion does occur it's usually after the patient has gone home, which means she'll go to the emergency room closest to her house, not the place her provider might have privileges.)

The second reason people on both sides of the issue knew these regulations weren't about health was the fact they reduced access to abortion. When the admitting privileges requirement went into effect, about half the abortion clinics in Texas closed because local hospitals refused to give clinic doctors admitting privileges. Clinic closures don't prove a law is bad—whether facilities do colonoscopies, knee surgeries, or abortions, unsafe outpatient clinics should be closed until they improve. It's the lack of evidence that Texas abortion clinics were unsafe, or that these regulations would make safe clinics even safer, that made the law's impact of clinic closures relevant. Hospitals often require a doctor to admit a minimum number of patients a year in order to receive admitting privileges. Because abortion is so safe, physicians who perform abortions never meet that minimum number of patients needing hospital care. And hospitals regularly refuse to give qualified physicians working in abortion clinics admitting privileges as a professional courtesy to avoid becoming embroiled in abortion politics.

So what was the real reason for the Texas law? To paraphrase James Carville, "It's the fetus, stupid." But Trojan Horse abortion laws don't say reducing the number of women who can obtain abortions is their goal. Instead they are packaged as regulations that protect patients.

In 2016 the U.S. Supreme Court reviewed the Texas law. In some ways, *Whole Woman's Health v. Hellerstedt* was a standard regulatory case. Except it was about abortion, so there was nothing "standard" about it. The lower court presumed courts can hear arguments about whether a statute does what the legislature claims it will. After reviewing the evidence, the lower court concluded that "[m]any of the building standards mandated by the act and its implementing rules have such a tangential relationship to patient safety in the context of abortion as to be nearly arbitrary," and ruled the Texas law was an unconstitutional burden (an "undue burden") on the abortion right.

The appellate court took the opposite position: courts must defer to a statute's stated purpose. The Texas legislature said the purpose of holding abortion clinics to ASC standards and requiring admitting privileges "was to provide the highest quality of care". Therefore, because there's always "medical uncertainty" about outcomes, the appellate court ruled the lower court "erred by substituting its own judgment for that of the legislature . . . ."

The U.S. Supreme Court ruled the lower court was correct in a 5–3 opinion written by Justice Breyer. (There were only eight sitting Justices at the time.) There was no charged rhetoric about women or fetuses. The decision simply affirmed that courts have "an independent constitutional duty to review factual findings where constitutional rights are at stake." Then it summarized the evidence, and because all the evidence showed the law would not improve health and safety, the Court struck down the Texas requirements as an "undue burden" on the abortion right.

Whole Woman's Health is significant because it's only the third time the U.S. Supreme Court has found an abortion regulation to be an undue burden.* However, the idea that legislatures will honestly state the goals of the laws they pass, and that if they don't, courts may evaluate the actual facts to protect Americans' exercise of their constitutional rights, seems like something citizens should have been able to take for granted before this. The fact the Supreme Court's ruling in *Whole Woman's Health* was considered a big win for the pro-choice camp is emblematic of just how embattled the abortion right is.

"Well, that's just how abortion politics go," some say. But there's something bigger going on.

* The first was in *Casey,* when the Court struck a spousal notification requirement as an undue burden. The second was the first time the Court reviewed a "partial birth" abortion ban. In *Stenberg v. Carhart* (2000), it ruled that the Nebraska ban was an undue burden because it also included the more common D&E procedure. However, as discussed in Chapter 2, in 2007 the Court approved the revised ban passed by Congress.

In the 1980s, there was a dramatic rise in anti-abortion activism. Historian Johanna Schoen describes this period in her book *Abortion After Roe*: "[I]n the 1970s most clinics experienced only the occasional group of picketers," but in the early 1980s, anti-abortion activists "grew frustrated and impatient with ineffective electoral and lobbying strategies." In 1984 there was a rash of clinic bombings, and things changed.

> Across the country, protesters began to adopt more aggressive picketing techniques. … Protesters accosted women entering abortion clinics, blocked their access, confronted them physically and verbally, followed them, traced license plate numbers, called their homes, entered clinics and disrupted procedures, poured glue into front door locks, picketed the homes of abortion providers and clinic personnel, sent threatening letters, and made threatening phone calls. … Administrators at clinics across the country reported that on some days they counted as many as 100 protesters in front of their clinics. Even when the numbers were much smaller, protesters were aggressive and disruptive.

Operation Rescue was formed in the mid-1980s, and its "protests transformed the antiabortion movement. Their clinic sit-ins and blockades drew hundreds of protesters from across the country." By the late 1980s these sit-ins were "the most important form of political expression of the antiabortion movement." For example, busloads of anti-abortion activists brought by Operation Rescue from across the country blocked access to Atlanta's abortion clinics for four consecutive months in 1988. During six weeks in Wichita in 1991, an Operation Rescue siege led to the arrest of 2,700 protesters. The staff of one clinic was barricaded in for 36 hours, and all three clinics in the city had to be temporarily closed.

Then things changed. "By the late 1980s, public opinion was slowly turning against the clinic sit-ins, as originally favorable media coverage began to focus on the shoving, grabbing, and screaming matches in front of abortion clinics and journalists depicted [Operation Rescue] members as the victimizers in this struggle," Schoen writes. The dramatic blockades of the 1980s and early 1990s ended because "the chaotic events in front of clinics increased the discomfort of more moderate antiabortion activists, who disliked the emotional tone and cult-like atmosphere of many of the sit-ins. By 1990, many moderate activists had ceased participation."*

In 1994, Congress passed the FACE Act ("Freedom of Access to Clinic Entrances"), and the Department of Justice created a Task Force on violence against abortion providers. The larger pro-life movement distanced itself from clinic-based "rescues" and Operation Rescue become less prominent.

Then came the flood of state laws restricting abortion. By 2000, 13 states had four or five types of abortion restrictions. Ten years later, 22 states had abortion restrictions, and the number of restrictions per state increased—five of these states had six or more restrictions. In 2016 alone, 18 states enacted 50 new abortion restrictions. By 2016, 26 states had enough restrictions that the Guttmacher

* Many abortion clinics are still picketed. For example, Dr. Willie Parker reports he's worked in eleven clinics in his career, and he has "never, ever—not once—entered my workplace without being verbally assaulted and harassed by people who see it as their God-given role to interfere with me and my work, and to question my Christian faith and the judgment of my patients" (*Life's Work*, 124–125). Schoen's observation is that the intensity and breadth of these protests changed dramatically when public opinion turned and the "moderate antiabortion activists" withdrew their support. However, in 2017, about a hundred people from different states (including the National Director of the group formerly known as Operation Rescue, now called Operation Save America) came to protest a clinic in Louisville, Kentucky, and they blocked the door. Some fear that cues from the Trump administration are encouraging the return of this blockade style of protest. "The Descent of Anti-Choice Radicals on Louisville Is a Preview of Protests to Come." *Rewire*, May 15, 2017, by Jessica Mason Pieklo, https://rewire.news/article/2017/05/15/anti-choice-radicals-louisville-preview-protests-come/.

Institute classified four of them as "hostile to abortion rights" and 22 of them as "extremely hostile."

Collectively, these hundreds of state laws make it difficult for women to exercise their constitutional rights, and they demean and degrade women who do so. The Texas law litigated in *Whole Woman's Health* is representative of a type of regulation that advocates call TRAP laws: "Targeted Regulation of Abortion Providers." TRAP laws burden clinics and providers in an attempt to eliminate or reduce their ability to provide care. The provider-oriented Trojan Horse laws hijack the critical concept of patient safety for their exterior. A second type of abortion regulation burdens patients in an attempt to eliminate or reduce their ability to seek care, and/or to punishing them for obtaining it. The patient-oriented Trojan Horse laws hijack concepts from bioethics, like informed decisionmaking, for their exterior.*

These disparate regulations have a singular purpose: continuing the campaign of the aggressive anti-abortion activists of the 1980s in a way that's palatable to moderates. On the outside, they look like "compromise"—something any reasonable person should welcome, or at least begrudgingly let inside. Inside these laws is an aggressive attack on a constitutional right. Understanding this legal onslaught as a "civilized" version of clinic assaults helps us understand the Trojan Horse trend as a subterfuge to end legal abortion by making it inaccessible.

To illustrate how the Trojan Horse trend moves the Operation Rescue agenda from the sidewalk to the inside of a doctor's office through force of law, let's consider patient-oriented Trojan Horse laws such as state-scripted "informed consent" speeches, forced

* The next wave of regulations is being framed as the state showing its "respect" for embryos and fetuses—for example, rules that make tissue disposal after abortion so difficult and expensive it could close clinics.

ultrasound viewing, and waiting periods. Here are three examples of how the Trojan Horse trend works:

1) *Anti-abortion message through "informed consent."* Protesters outside abortion clinics often shout their opinion of the moral status of embryos and fetuses at patients, and sometimes offer patients "sidewalk counseling." ("In general, sidewalk counselors were to inform patients of the alleged dangers of abortion and the stages of fetal development in hopes that women might, at the last minute, change their mind about abortion." Schoen 172.)

As of 2017, 29 states force doctors to give state-scripted "informed consent" speeches before abortion. Six states require doctors to tell their patients personhood begins at conception, five require doctors to assert a false link between abortion and increased risk of breast cancer, four require doctors to give false information about abortion and risk to future fertility, and twenty-eight include information on fetal development throughout pregnancy. Protesters in these states can stay home, knowing the state is delivering their message to patients by forcing clinic staff to say it for them.

2) *Anti-abortion imagery through "informed consent."* Protesters outside abortion clinics often show patients photographs of fetuses. ("[D]emonstrators walked up and down the public sidewalk, praying and carrying signs with large photographs of mutilated fetuses" at a clinic in Philadelphia. Schoen 173.)

As of 2017, 26 states regulated the use of ultrasound in abortion clinics. Four of them force doctors to show patients her embryo or fetus's image and describe it before she may proceed with her abortion.

(That number was six, until two such laws were struck by courts.[*]) Protesters in these states can stay home, knowing the state is making clinic staff put a medicalized version of their sidewalk posters in women's faces for them.

3) *Clinic blockade through waiting periods.* Protesters' ultimate goal is to keep women away from abortion clinics, and in the 1980s, protests and bomb threats sometimes caused clinics to close temporarily. A secondary goal is to shame those who do go in. ("Some clients entered the clinic crying and shaking, while others—too frightened to confront the crowd of screaming demonstrators—asked to be rescheduled or referred to another clinic" during the Atlanta protests of 1988. Schoen 193.)

As of 2017, 27 states have waiting periods, which keep women away from abortion for 18 to 72 hours after their informed consent conversation. (Fourteen states require women to make two trips to the same clinic; other states allow the information to be given over the phone.)

* The federal appellate court that struck this provision in the North Carolina "Woman's Right to Know Act" concluded it was compelled speech that violated the First Amendment rights of doctors. The Court reasoned that the state's goal was "to use the visual imagery of the fetus to dissuade the patient from continuing with the planned procedure ... [which is] ideological; it conveys a particular opinion. ... Transforming the physician into the mouthpiece of the state undermines the trust that is necessary for facilitating healthy doctor-patient relationships and, through them, successful treatment outcomes." *Stuart v. Camnitz*, 774 F.3d 238 (4th Cir. 2014), 245, 253, *cert. denied*, 135 S. Ct. 2838 (2015). However, two years earlier the same federal appellate court that deferred to the legislature's stated intent in *Whole Woman's Health* found a similar section of the Texas "Woman's Right to Know Act" was not impermissibly compelled ideological speech: "The point of informed consent laws is to allow the patient to evaluate her condition and render her best decision under difficult circumstances. Denying her up to date medical information is more of an abuse to her ability to decide than providing the information." *Texas Med. Providers v. Lakey*, 667 F.3d 570, 579 (5th Cir. 2012). (Oklahoma is the second state where a law like this was struck; that state court ruled on different grounds. *Nova Health Systems v. Pruitt*, 2012 OK 103, 292 P.3d 28 (Okla. 2012) (per curiam).)

Laws requiring women to wait to receive a procedure they've been informed about and have decided they want simultaneously shame them and delay their abortions, factors I consider in more detail below. Protesters in these states can stay home, knowing the state is disrupting women's ability to access abortion clinics for them.*

History enriches our understanding of the Trojan Horse trend. Sociology can take it another step, broadening the way we understand this legal trend to include institutional policy and social practice, all of which contribute to structural stigma.

When sociologists introduced the concept of stigma in the 1960s, stigma was thought of as something conveyed or enforced through individual interactions. Imagine a white woman named Agnes muttering a racial slur at an African-American woman named Harriet as they pass. That's an example of the original understanding of stigma.

More recently, sociologists have developed the concept of structural stigma. Professors Bruce Link and Jo Phelan explain that structural stigma is a system of laws, institutional policies, and cultural norms that limit the opportunities, resources, and well-being of the stigmatized. Examples of structural stigma include laws requiring racially segregated schools, institutional policies of private banks that led to racially discriminatory loan practices, and a social norm that forbade whites and African-Americans from eating together. Structural stigma is often more efficient and thorough than stigma conveyed through direct personal interaction. Individual stigmatizers can't be everywhere, and structural stigma relieves them of the burden or embarrassment of person-to-person discrimination.

A "Whites Only" sign above a drinking fountain is an example of structural stigma. This sign relieves Agnes of the effort (and the risk)

* TRAP laws that regulate clinics out of existence or affordability obviously accomplish the goal of delaying or denying access as well.

of insulting Harriet to her face. Instead, the state communicates the message that Harriet is a second-class citizen to Harriet on Agnes's behalf through the sign, and it keeps doing it after Agnes has gone home.

When a system of structural stigma achieves Agnes's aims at the macro level, not only can Agnes behave as if she is not racist, she can *believe* she is not racist. When Agnes's sense of racial order is enforced by laws, institutions, and cultural norms, she doesn't even have to admit her feelings of racial superiority privately to herself. As Link and Phelan (who apply this theory to the politics of mental health) observe, "Things work more smoothly for stigmatizers if their interests are misrecognized by others and themselves such that they are either not observed at all or judged to be just the natural order of things."

"Self-stigma" can result from structural stigma that makes inferiority seem "just the natural order of things," instead of just one hateful person or group's opinion. Internalizing negative social stereotypes of African-Americans can lead Harriet to believe and act as if they are true. Self-stigma can ultimately result in the insidious effect of self-policing. People don't chafe at oppression and challenge preconceptions after they internalize negative assessments of their group. Instead, they "stay in their place." Structural stigma accomplishes the stigmatizers' goals by keeping the targeted group *in* (within social norms), *down* (dominating or exploiting them to gain power, wealth, or social status), and *away* (isolating those who do violate the norm, and inducing others to isolate them on an individual level).

Earlier I mentioned waiting periods as a legislative version of an aggressive protest tactic. Let's go back and look at waiting periods through the lens of structural stigma. At first glance, state laws forcing women to wait one to three days between abortion counseling and having the procedure might seem like a minor imposition—just the state saying "let's take this decision seriously," and who disagrees with that? And she still gets to have the abortion. So aren't waiting periods a reasonable compromise?

After a woman finds out she's pregnant, at some point she makes a doctor's appointment. Whether that's for prenatal care or pregnancy termination, her phone call is the culmination of a thought process, not the beginning. Perhaps that's why, in a nationally representative survey, 92% of women obtaining abortions said they had made up their mind before they made their abortion appointment. Some women know whether or not they want to have a child long before they learn they're pregnant. For others, the plus sign on the pee stick might be what prompts them to think through their values, desires, and circumstances (whether alone or in discussion with partner, family, friends, or clergy) in order to decide which doctor to call. But 92% reflects what common sense would suggest—most thinking about parenthood is more likely to happen at home than in a doctor's office.*

Some women who call for an abortion appointment change their minds and don't show up. As one of the leading textbooks for training abortion counselors puts it, "Most women who arrive for their abortion appointments are sure that abortion is the best decision for them

* Abortion is a constitutional right one can't exercise without the help of a medical professional. As a result, all abortion is health care. Yet like delivering a baby in a hospital, the fact abortion usually has to happen in a medical setting to be safe doesn't mean it's *only* a medical event. "Abortion is exclusively a medical decision" could be considered a masterplot that *Roe* helped create by anchoring the abortion right in the social authority of physicians. Some abortions I'm calling "extraordinary" fit the traditional medical decisionmaking model perfectly: when a woman must weigh complex medical information about how much and how certainly pregnancy threatens her health, or an anomaly or disease threatens her fetus's health, against the benefits of continuing her wanted pregnancy, medical facts will play a central role in her abortion decisionmaking. Yet in both extraordinary and ordinary abortion, a woman who has decided she doesn't want to continue her pregnancy is unlikely to change her mind based on the medical facts of the procedure used to accomplish her goal, just as a pregnant woman who has decided she wants to deliver a baby is unlikely to change her mind based on the medical facts of childbirth. As a result, a unique need to think about the abortion procedure itself cannot possibly justify waiting periods.

at this time in their lives. If they are really unsure or have decided that they want to continue the pregnancy, they often won't come to their appointment. For some, making an appointment and then 'no-showing' is an important part of the decision-making process." Abortion counselors then assess the certainty of the decision of those who have indicated their desire by making an appointment and coming to that appointment. Those who arrive conflicted or ambivalent about whether they want to have a baby (whether to parent or for adoption), or who want to discuss a difficult decision to not have a baby, are likely to benefit from in-depth counseling. But like all quality care, that's not a one-size-fits-all speech, it's tailored to the individual patient. (To return to the "informed consent" point for a moment: Imagine if your state required all obstetricians providing prenatal care to give every happy woman who comes to them a state-scripted speech saying her odds of dying while delivering a baby are approximately fourteen times higher than if she had an abortion, 10–20% of new mothers suffer from postpartum depression, and P.S., here's the insane amount of money college will cost in eighteen years, so go home and think about this baby thing a little longer. The accuracy of these facts doesn't cure the underlying insult.)

Those who defend waiting periods make a simple suggestion: Shouldn't a woman having an abortion think about it for at least a day? Sure. But why would you assume she hasn't? Waiting periods send women who've chosen abortion a degrading message: your state thinks you are so stupid that the first moment you would consider the consequences of ending your pregnancy is the moment you consented to a medical procedure that does exactly that. Instead of being treated as an adult who is wise enough to assess whether she's ready to act after that counseling conversation, the legislature thinks you need a toddler's time out to think about what you said. They insult physicians similarly: your state thinks you are so despicable that if a patient expressed uncertainty in the consent process, instead of suggesting she come back if and when she's certain, you would herd her through for an abortion anyway. Seen through the historical lens of the goals and actions of groups like Operation Rescue, and through the sociological lens of structural stigma, laws that require every woman seeking an abortion to wait, regardless of how certain she is or how long she considered the decision before making the appointment, are better understood as delay laws.

In addition to emotional and psychological burdens, structural stigma creates practical burdens. Delay laws can require some women to travel to faraway clinics twice, or to pay hotel expenses to stay in that town for the duration of the delay. Delay laws can mean missing more work or having to find more child care, and more difficulty finding someone who will accompany you if the procedure requires sedation. The added expense of overcoming these obstacles functions as an abortion tax, increasing the total cost of exercising a constitutional right. The time it takes some women to raise that money can delay their abortion, which can also increase the procedure's expense.

The clinic assaults of the 1980s and early 1990s that made the "more moderate anti-abortion activists" Schoen describes uncomfortable are now codified, civilized, and institutionalized in a way that this group either supports or ignores. (It's possible the same is true of "more moderate" abortion supporters—those who want legality, but are ambivalent about abortion's morality.)

Yet Trojan Horse abortion laws are arguably more stigmatizing than clinic blockades. They get inside the clinic, forcing physicians and counselors to deliver the protesters' message for them. They give an anti-abortion message that used to be attributable to private individuals the imprimatur of the government. And they have the added benefit of freeing individual stigmatizers to spend the time and energy they would have invested in clinic blockades on more enjoyable things.

So far I have focused on law. However, the concept of structural stigma illuminates the fact that sometimes law isn't needed to keep physicians and patients from abortion care. Institutional policies and social practices can do it just as effectively.

A former student heard I was pregnant and invited me to lunch to talk birthing and babies. Since I'd last seen her, Dr. Penelope Lasalle had finished a prestigious residency in obstetrics and gynecology and she'd had two children, but she was still the chatty funny young woman I remembered from class. When Dr. Lasalle interviewed for her first job in private practice, she asked if in addition to delivering babies in hospitals and doing routine gynecological care in the office, she could also do early surgical abortions, or at least offer medication abortion for her patients, as an integrated part of her office practice. The physician who owned the group said no. Why? "I don't want to be known as the practice in town that does that."

Listening to Dr. Lasalle's story, I was struck by how closely it fit a pattern documented by sociologist Lori Freedman in her book *Willing and Unable*. One study of ob/gyns found that before residency 33% of those surveyed intended to provide abortions, but only half that group ended up doing so. To better understand why, Professor Freedman interviewed ob/gyns practicing across the country who trained in residency programs like Dr. Lasalle's, which provide abortion training unless residents choose to opt out. Only one in Freedman's sample who wanted to integrate abortion into private practice had been able to do so. The others were stopped, not by laws, but by social and professional costs and constraints "born of the stigma and politics of abortion for which American medicine has proved a weak adversary."

At lunch Dr. Lasalle told me she'd "be happy" to include abortion in her private practice. Yet she took the job that prohibited her from doing so. Later I asked to interview her to understand why.

Dr. Lasalle's first reason was personal: she and her husband wanted jobs near their families so their relatives could help with child care. Child care was a major consideration for the physicians Freedman interviewed as well—her sample was ob/gyns five to ten years out of residency, and the need to live near extended family limited geographic options for many. Dr. Lasalle's second reason was professional: she's trained to do a broad range of office gynecology and hospital obstetric procedures, and this breadth is what she loves about her specialty. She'd be willing to do a little moonlighting at Planned Parenthood as a way of keeping abortion in her practice, but her employment contract prohibits her from working anywhere else while employed in the practice. This too is consistent with Freedman's findings: "[T]hose wanting to include abortion in their [private] practices often have an unsatisfying choice to make: either practice obstetrics and gynecology *or* provide abortions, but not both."

When we spoke, Dr. Lasalle had been working with her practice group for two years, but she had felt no need to challenge their restrictions. Why? Because there's a Planned Parenthood twenty minutes from her office. She thinks Planned Parenthood takes good care of her patients (she doesn't see any problems in the emergency room when she's covering obstetric emergencies, or in her patients with abortions in their medical history), and its presence means her patients rarely ask her to do their abortions (she mostly treats educated wealthy women who diagnose unwanted pregnancy at home and know to go to Planned Parenthood). Because Dr. Lasalle doesn't feel there's an unmet need for abortion in her suburb, she sees little benefit to fighting to change her practice owner's policy.

But she does see a cost: the financial cost of losing patients. "The [physician] group would worry that patients wouldn't go to a doctor or group that did terminations. I'm not sure that's true, but it is a conservative suburb." Is it possible she'd gain as many pro-choice patients as she'd lose? "I don't think it would balance out. I don't think there would be patients who seek out a practice that does terminations just to support it. But there would be patients who leave to show their opposition."

Many people know that some religiously affiliated hospitals refuse to participate in abortions except to save the pregnant woman's life. However, policies that make abortion care more difficult to obtain also exist in secular (non-religious) institutions. The hospital where Dr. Lasalle's private practice group does 95% of their out-of-office procedures is a secular community hospital with no religious affiliation. Yet it too has an explicit policy that elective abortions cannot be performed there. When Dr. Lasalle was hired, the owner later added that one physician in their private group had a religious objection to abortion. The policies of this secular hospital and Dr. Lasalle's employer are consistent with Freedman's finding that physicians practicing in groups often created anti-abortion policies to avoid conflict. If one physician in the group was uncomfortable with abortion, no physician in the group was allowed to provide it.

On one hand, this is a nice show of respect. I care deeply about religious liberty, and I'd like everyone to be comfortable too. On the other hand, it's an odd form of hostage-taking. Social norms around abortion care mean an individual or a minority is often allowed to constrain the behavior of the majority of health care providers in the group, and patients have no voice in these negotiations.

Dr. Lasalle's practice group and the hospital they use would have to change their policies for her to include abortion in her practice, and she's "not willing to fight that battle." But she was adamant that if her patients were not getting good abortion care from whoever was providing it, or if she lived in a state where she had no nearby place to refer them to, "that would be a whole different story." I would like to think Dr. Lasalle would be the exception, but in Freedman's study, obstetricians like her who moved to small towns where their services were most needed felt too vulnerable to provide abortions. On the other end of the spectrum, those working in urban settings, like Dr. Lasalle, shared her assessment. They felt their patients had plenty of safe options, so they saw little benefit in exchange for the social penalty they might experience for providing the service.

I've always been fond of Dr. Lasalle. I respect the investment she made to become a doctor, and I think she deserves a safe, profitable, satisfying professional life. The problem is, I feel the same way about the physicians I've never met who work at her local Planned Parenthood. These doctors endure the penalties thousands of physicians avoid—penalties that are greater than they would be if they were spread among a larger number of doctors providing abortion care. By providing access to safe abortion, the doctors and nurses who do abortions make the satisfying professional lives of thousands of ob/gyns like Dr. Lasalle possible—lives in which they avoid the abortion controversy, *and* sleep well at night knowing their patients can end unwanted pregnancies safely.

Talking with Dr. Lasalle made me realize that the structural stigma that shapes the delivery of American abortion care has created another, rarely recognized group of beneficiaries: all the physicians, nurses, hospital administrators, and other health care workers who would be personally devastated to see women harmed by unsafe abortion, and who could provide this service themselves, but choose not to. Like men who benefit from their girlfriend's choice to have an abortion, these clinicians benefit from their colleagues' choice to provide abortion.

As Freedman puts it, "[m]any physicians want both distance from abortion and someone skilled to send their patients to." As Dr. Lasalle puts it, "This is problematic thinking, I know. Sometimes I get conflicted."

Bioethics considers how doctors should take care of patients. The politics of abortion requires us to expand that analysis to consider how medical professionals should take care of one another in order to preserve the well-being of their shared patients. The same patients ask allergists, orthopedic surgeons, physicians and nurses who provide abortions, internists, and ophthalmologists for health care at different points in their lives. To maintain their own patients' safety and health, more clinicians in every other medical specialty should offer concrete, compensatory support to those who shoulder the burden of providing their patients' abortion care.

Structural stigma is created by social norms as well. Christopher Lapin is a full-time ethics consultant at an institution I'll call Midwestern Hospital. An ethics consultant is a person some hospitals have on staff to help with individual cases raising thorny ethical problems, and to contribute to hospital policy. Mr. Lapin is a wiry man with a brown mustache, tweedy jackets, and an earnest energy, and after I gave a paper at a bioethics conference, he volunteered that his hospital's obstetrics department had reached what he described as a "détente" on abortion cases. Midwestern Hospital is an academic medical center that also doesn't do "elective" abortions; it only does abortions for "medical indications," meaning a problem with the health of a woman or her embryo or fetus. Yet unlike every other obstetrics case, instead of being assigned to these patients, medical staff are asked to affirmatively volunteer. It can take 24 to 48 hours to schedule a full team of willing participants (anesthesiologist, nurses, residents, etcetera) together in an open operating room—so staffing these cases created lots of anxiety, but care was delivered. Then the détente collapsed. At my request, Mr. Lapin later told me the full story of structural stigma as social practice at Midwestern Hospital.

In the election season of 2012, the local political climate around abortion became particularly rancorous. People at the hospital followed suit, becoming "blunt, coarse, and forceful" in how they talked about abortion. At the same time, changes in state law that stopped other facilities from doing abortions increased the volume of abortion cases at Midwestern Hospital.

Nurses who opposed abortion began refusing to answer the call lights of abortion patients. They sabotaged patient care by doing things like agreeing to put in an order for an abortion patient then not doing so, or agreeing to adjust their schedule and then switching back at the last minute. They ostracized the nurses who did care for the hospital's abortion patients, giving them the silent treatment in common areas. And they put their colleagues in one of two categories, openly calling them part of either "the baby killers" or "the Christians." "The work environment had become beyond hostile," the ethicist said. As the pressure rose, fewer and fewer staff were volunteering to care for patients receiving abortions. Residents (young doctors finishing their training) who were distressed that these nurses were inhibiting their ability to provide medical care called the ethicist for help.

Mr. Lapin began by speaking to many staff members in the unit. He found "[a] few very loud, fervent people" opposed abortion, a dwindling small number participated in the cases, and a large number were "in the middle. ... They were ambivalent and unsure about how they felt about [abortion], and as long as somebody else was willing to do it they were happy to opt out. So they wouldn't necessarily volunteer for it, but they'd be willing to do it if push came to shove." Another issue was that some of the saboteurs were in positions of power. "Because leaders knew what was going on, [those who were bullied] weren't getting support. That's what I finally uncovered, that the nursing leadership was stealthily undermining any opportunity to create a healthy work environment."

To further educate himself about the situation, the ethicist followed a woman having a second-trimester abortion through her two days of hospital care. "She was Catholic. Her priest supported her. In her mind, every time they did an ultrasound they found a new problem with her baby. She referred to it as her baby, not the fetus. So in her mind she was preventing suffering." The ethicist was relieved to see this patient got excellent care. "[T]he people on staff who were willing to take care of her were unbelievably amazing. ... I have incredible respect for the people who are willing to do that in an environment where it's clear there are people who do not support what they do, and if given the opportunity would make their lives miserable." He was particularly moved by one of the residents who was upset about the nurses' obstruction. "[H]e was from Egypt, and he said 'I'm learning this procedure because I know this will save women's lives when I go home. And these people here don't have a clue about what women face.'"

A clinician himself, the ethicist was shocked at how the professionalism of the medical workplace went out the window when the topic was abortion. "This is unacceptable from a nursing standpoint in any way." The gravity of the situation led him to involve a senior hospital administrator. Together they hosted a departmental meeting to clarify hospital policy, which says clinicians may morally object to a procedure, but they cannot object to a person or class of patient. Their primary message was "to remind them, first and foremost, that [the hospital's] values are centered on respect, and whether or not you disagree with someone, you have to respect them."

What happened at Midwestern Hospital? The ethicist had an interesting take on it:

> People had lost the ability to demand the respect of others. People were being bullied, and they let themselves be bullied. I know that sounds bad, but they didn't have the tools to stop the bullying. ... We don't give people the language they need to respond. Because it's not socially acceptable to *advocate* for abortion. It's one thing to accept it. It's another thing to advocate for it. ... [I]f people can be given the language to help them to be at peace with a decision they know they need to make or a stance they know they need to take it's much easier to be present with people who are against it.

In abortion care, a climate in which health care providers accommodate colleagues who oppose abortion, but no accommodation flows the other way, is one of polite discrimination. On an institutional level, employees using conscience as a club raises organizational ethics issues, such as fidelity to missions of patient care or education. On a social level, unreciprocal respect is a threat to pluralism. Normalizing it also paves the way for polite discrimination to transform into the kind of open hostility found at Midwestern Hospital.

The most extreme private expression of stigma is violence. Historian Schoen points out that the decline in enthusiasm for the dramatic clinic blockades and mass protests of the 1980s left splinter groups and radicalized individuals who "escalate[d] protests to a level of harassment and violence that, by the early 1990s, included the killing of abortion providers and staff working at abortion clinics."

Eleven people associated with abortion have been murdered by abortion opponents: Dr. David Gunn in 1993, Dr. John Bayard Britton and volunteer clinic escort James Barrett in 1994, Planned Parenthood receptionists Shannon Lowney and Leanne Nichols in 1994, Dr. Barnett Slepian in 1998, clinic security guard Robert Sanderson in 1998, Dr. George Tiller in 2009, and campus police officer Garrett Swasey and clinic patrons Ke'Arre M. Stewart and Jennifer Markovsky in 2015. Many more providers have been terrorized—for example, between 1977 and 2016 the National Abortion Federation (NAF), the professional organization of abortion providers, has recorded 26 attempted murders, 42 clinic bombings, and 185 acts of arson.*

Structural stigma creates a climate that encourages political violence—violence directed at an entire group through attacks on

* Sociologist Carole Joffe offers an accessible, compelling account of violence against people and places associated with abortion in *Dispatches from the Abortion Wars: The Costs of Fanaticism to Doctors, Patients, and the Rest of Us* (Beacon Press, 2011).

individual members. Physical attacks on people associated with abortion clinics have some things in common with lynching—extraordinary events singling out people who violated Jim Crow etiquette or exercised their civil rights. This targeted violence reinforced the laws, institutional policies, and social norms preserving white dominance. Violence against some African-Americans reminded every African-American what the consequences could be if they didn't stay in, down, and away. Violence against abortion providers does something similar. At one level we deplore it. At another level we accept it as normal, because "abortion is like that." But it doesn't have to be. Those who reject violence should reject the structural stigma that facilitates it.

The concept of structural stigma highlights how abuse can be inflicted without any individual person insulting or assaulting another. In some places, it's through law. In other places, it's through a quiet understanding of economics or a desire to avoid social conflict in the workplace that leads to institutional policies keeping trained physicians who are willing to provide abortion away from patients. In other places, the malevolence of abortion politics is allowed to poison the professionalism of medical practice. Silence in the face of Jim Crow was not an apolitical stance on race relations. The same is true today with "Jane Crow" abortion laws, private policies, and social practices.

It would be ridiculous to suggest that 21st-century abortion law is exactly the same as the Jim Crow system of racial segregation. Jim Crow attacked African-Americans in multiple areas of their lives, throughout their lives, on the basis of an immutable and visible characteristic. In contrast, today some women live in a general climate of opportunity and respect until they are attacked on the basis of one action (although the ability to become pregnant is an aspect of the immutable characteristic of gender), and those who join the group of "women who have had abortions" can usually hide their membership if they want to. Similarly, lynchings (which were often accompanied by torture and mutilation) were often witnessed, cheered on, and photographed by large groups of people, and that is very different in fact and message than shootings by lone gunmen.

My point is simply that the distance that allows us to see the forest of one discriminatory system could help us navigate a different set of trees we're lost among today. As Link and Phelan put it, "[m]isrecognition serves the interests of the powerful because it allows their interests to be achieved surreptitiously." Anti-abortion laws quietly justify and generate private polices and social norms that also decrease respect, autonomy, and access to quality heath care for women. That's why understanding Trojan Horse abortion laws for what they are is a precursor to improving the American abortion conversation.

II. RUSSIAN DOLLS

Trojan Horse abortion laws hide an argument about the moral status of embryos and fetuses. For some people, the agenda ends there.

For others, the more accurate image might be a Russian Doll. Nested inside an argument about embryonic and fetal status is a hidden argument about the proper role of women. Inside that might be an argument about the proper role of sex ... or the proper role of religion in governance ... or a fear white people aren't reproducing enough to stay on top ... and so on.

The Russian Doll problem is one of both clarity and sincerity. Hidden agendas muddy the American abortion debate. The social conflicts that have taken up residence inside the topic of abortion are thoroughly discussed in many places. However, openly identifying them in any given exchange could help us clarify what we're actually talking about. Sincerity becomes an issue when these other agendas are intentionally hidden. Some pro-choice people would like to be in dialogue with honest abolitionists—abortion opponents with no agenda other than a heartfelt conviction that it's wrong to end embryonic life. But the difficulty of distinguishing honest abolitionists from people who oppose abortion because they're opposed to women's sexual freedom, or women's new social and economic roles, or other hidden concerns, and an unwillingness to be suckered into earnest conversation on false premises, can lead pro-choice people to avoid conversation about the moral value of embryos and fetuses altogether.

The social agendas hidden inside the Russian Doll of abortion are another reason the fight on this topic has continued. Abortion isn't just philosophically complex. Abortion is threatening.

When Sylvia Law began law school in 1965, she was one of only 21 women in a class of 300. Seven percent was the highest proportion ever, and even that peak was in part because many potential male law students avoided the war in Vietnam by doing public service. After the holiday break, class ranking by first-semester grades was posted on a bulletin board, and seven of the top ten people in the class were women. Sylvia was studying the list, happy to learn she was in the top 3% of the class, when the director of admissions joined her in reviewing it. Sylvia commented that the women had done well. "Sylvia, this is not good for the girls," he responded. "We need those top places for people who will go on to bring money and honor to the school. You know these girls aren't going to do that."

It's easy to forget that the idea women have value outside the domestic sphere of home and family is relatively new. But for the first 144 years of America's existence, women weren't allowed to vote. Almost a hundred years after a constitutional amendment changed that in 1920, in 2017 the U.S. Congress was only 19% female. In contrast, Sylvia's law school admission in 1965 is a marker of the rapid advances women have made in higher education and the professions in only a few decades.

In 1870 the Illinois Supreme Court denied the application of Mrs. Myra Bradwell for a license to practice law on the grounds that although she was qualified, the law did not allow married women to enter into their own contracts, which practicing lawyers must do. The U.S. Supreme Court affirmed the denial, and the opinion of three concurring Justices summarizes the "two spheres" philosophy:

> [T]he civil law, as well as nature herself, has always recognized a wide difference in the respective spheres and destinies of man and woman. … The Constitution of the family organization, which is founded in the divine ordinance as well as in the nature of things, indicates the domestic sphere as that which properly belongs to the domain and functions of womanhood. The harmony, not to say identity, of interest and views which belong, or should belong, to the family institution is repugnant to the idea of a woman adopting a distinct and independent career from that of her husband. So firmly fixed was this sentiment in the founders of the common law that it became a maxim of that system of jurisprudence that a woman had no legal existence separate from her husband. … The paramount destiny and mission of woman are to fulfill the noble and benign offices of wife and mother. This is the law of the Creator. And the rules of civil society must be adapted to the general constitution of things, and cannot be based upon exceptional cases.

A hundred years after Mrs. Bradwell's application was rejected, in 1970, only 8% of law students were women. Ten years later that number more than quadrupled—in 1980, 34% of law students were women. In 2011, women accounted for almost half of all law degrees, and in 2013 over one-third of practicing attorneys were women. This change in my field is representative of a dramatic gender shift in the American workforce generally.

Five years after Sylvia finished law school, the Supreme Court decided *Roe v. Wade*. In those years Sylvia was working with poor women on rights to obtain basic subsistence and health care on equal and dignified terms, and future Justice Ruth Bader Ginsburg was fighting for gender equality in public service and employment and the right of women to keep their jobs when they became pregnant in her role as the founding head of the ACLU's Women's Rights Project. Neither of these lawyers was deeply involved in the early legal struggles for reproductive rights. However, working for equal rights for women in the public sphere led them to see a different rationale for the constitutional protection of abortion. In 1973, *Roe v. Wade* anchored abortion in a constitutional right to privacy. In 1984, Law and Ginsburg each independently concluded that reproductive freedom should be treated not as a privacy right, but as an issue of constitutionally protected gender equality. As Sylvia put it, abortion bans "raise equality concerns because state control of a woman's reproductive capacity and exaggeration of the significance of biological difference has historically been central to the oppression of women," and "an equality doctrine that denies the reality of biological difference in relation to reproduction reflects an idea about personhood that is inconsistent with people's actual experience of themselves and the world." *

More recently, legal scholar Reva Siegel has extended the gender equality analysis of abortion to the siege of Trojan Horse abortion laws discussed above. Siegel offers a blistering analysis of the recent rhetorical shift in abortion opposition. This shift drops the old focus on how abortion harms fetuses, and replaces it with a supposedly "pro-woman" claim that abortion harms women. Therefore, the

* Contrary to the prediction of the director of admissions, Sylvia did all right for NYU School of Law. In 1973 she became one of her alma mater's first female professors, and in 1983 she was the first lawyer in the United States to be awarded a MacArthur "genius grant."

current argument goes, women need to be protected from abortion, and they are the intended beneficiaries of anti-abortion laws. Siegel points out that this is the same "woman-protective" argument legislatures and courts have used for centuries to justify discriminatory laws keeping women from employment and civil life.

Women's sexuality is part of the equality equation in the private realm, and that's one reason issues of gender equality and sex are hard to separate. Women's ability to reliably do what men have been able to do for the approximately 200,000 years *Homo sapiens* has been around—enjoy sex without having a baby afterward—is relatively recent, and medical technologies giving women the option of breaking the link between sex and childbearing shift the balance of interpersonal power significantly.

Social anxiety about sex is usually limited to unmarried people, and until recently, pregnancy served as both disincentive to sex outside of marriage and evidence that it occurred. Yet America's low birth rate suggests that like single people, the intention of married couples' lovemaking is rarely reproductive. (The fact 14% of abortion patients are married also tells us that not every pregnancy within marriage is welcome.) Married people have sex for the same reasons unmarried people do—physical pleasure and emotional intimacy. For some, a couple's legal commitment to one another is what makes their lovemaking morally permissible. For others, the division is not just between unmarried and married sex, but between procreative and nonprocreative sex.

For example, in 1995 Pope John Paul II reiterated the Catholic doctrine that marital sex is always meant to be reproductive. The Catholic Church opposes contraception because it "contradicts the full truth of the sexual act as the proper expression of conjugal love" and contraception "is opposed to the virtue of chastity in marriage."

State governments used to enact this perspective on marital (and nonmarital) sex through law. The same year Sylvia started law school,

1965, the Supreme Court reviewed a case in which two Planned Parenthood employees were arrested for providing married women with contraception. In *Griswold v. Connecticut,* the Court ruled that a Connecticut law criminalizing the use or distribution of contraception violated a new doctrine that the Court articulated in this case: the right of privacy.

The Constitution doesn't mention contraception, but the Court recounted a long history of cases that looked beyond the text of different amendments to protect citizens from governmental intrusion that violated the spirit of those amendments. In prior cases, several parts of the Bill of Rights had been interpreted to protect different aspects of privacy. The Court identified marriage as "a relationship lying within the zone of privacy created by several fundamental constitutional guarantees. . . . We deal with a right of privacy older than the Bill of Rights," and held that Connecticut's ban on contraception was an unconstitutional intrusion on the intimate relationship between husband and wife.

After the *Griswold* ruling on the Connecticut law in 1965, Hester Prynne's home state of Massachusetts could have complied by repealing its own law criminalizing contraception. Instead, in 1966 it amended it to ban contraception only for unmarried people.

The Massachusetts contraceptive ban stemmed from an 1879 law prohibiting the distribution of contraceptives. In 1917, the state's highest court explained that the law's plain purpose was "to preserve chastity," but in *Eisenstadt v. Baird* (1972), the U.S. Supreme Court struggled to find a legitimate state interest for the Massachusetts ban on contraception for single people. The year before the Supreme Court ruled, a state court said the purpose of the legislation was to discourage premarital intercourse.* However, the U.S. Supreme Court asserted, "[i]t would be plainly unreasonable to assume that Massachusetts

* In 1971, a Massachusetts court reasoned that the phrase "intended to be used as contraceptives" in the law did not include contraceptives intended for prevention of disease. As a result, both single and married people could legally buy condoms, but it was still illegal

has prescribed pregnancy and the birth of an unwanted child as punishment for fornication," although "fornication" remained a misdemeanor. So the Court cut to the chase—since married people now had a constitutional right to contraception, state laws that criminalized the same act for single people violated the Equal Protection Clause: "If the right of privacy means anything, it is the right of the individual, married or single, to be free from unwarranted governmental intrusion into matters so fundamentally affecting a person as the decision whether to bear or beget a child." *

My students can't believe some states made it illegal to use contraception as late as the 1970s. They think of these laws as something from the Puritan era, and they have a hard time understanding why women's access to contraception required a fight. But the history of the contraception cases is important to those who pooh-pooh the possibility that some opposition to abortion is driven by anxiety about women having sex. It's also interesting to note that the "extraordinary abortions" many find compelling are the cases that don't suggest a woman had sex for (or only for) pleasure. Sex that was planned or accepted as procreative underlies abortions done for reasons of maternal or fetal health, and sex that doesn't meet typical standards of consent underlies abortions done for reasons of rape, incest, or extreme youth.

In the same influential 1995 Encyclical quoted above, Pope John Paul II acknowledged the shared goals of contraception and abortion. "[D]espite their differences of nature and moral gravity,

for women to get contraception they controlled, like the revolutionary new pharmaceutical called the Pill.

* In 1977, the Court extended the right to contraception to minors. In *Carey v. Population Services*, New York defended its law as furthering its "policy against promiscuous sexual intercourse among the young." Since New York could not prohibit a minor from ending an unwanted pregnancy with abortion, the Court reasoned that it could not constitutionally prohibit her from trying to prevent one.

contraception and abortion are often closely connected, as fruits of the same tree. … [Both] are rooted in a hedonistic mentality unwilling to accept responsibility in matters of sexuality, and they imply a self-centered concept of freedom, which regards procreation as an obstacle to personal fulfillment."*

The Supreme Court also saw a connection between contraception and abortion. The same connection that led the Pope to critique "the contraceptive mentality" led the Supreme Court to extend the privacy right it applied to contraception in *Griswold* and *Eisenstadt* to abortion in *Roe*. The contraception cases mean the state can't try to stop you from choosing to have nonprocreative sex by banning contraception. The abortion cases mean that if you do accidentally become pregnant, the state can't force you to have a child.

Abortion is not contraception. Contraception prevents pregnancy, and abortion ends pregnancy. Abortion *is* "birth control." People using contraception and people having abortions have the same goal: preventing birth. The dreaded "abortion as birth control" criticism usually refers to people who don't use contraception. That critique may have blinded us to a different conversation, which acknowledges the way abortion functions as Plan C (or D, or Z) for some contraceptive-using Americans. Both contraceptive use and ordinary abortion occur when women have sex because they want

* The current Pope has not changed this doctrine. This is important to the practice of medicine, because it means doctors working in Catholic health care facilities are still not allowed to prescribe contraception to prevent pregnancy even in married couples, perform vasectomy or tubal ligation, or end pregnancy through abortion (unless the pregnancy threatens the woman's life). The large market share of Catholic healthcare (one in every six acute care hospital beds in the U.S. is in a facility that is Catholic owned or affiliated) means this policy affects many patients of all (and no) faiths. Although Pope Francis has taken a more sympathetic tone, and he has given priests authority to forgive the sin of abortion (a power that was previously reserved for bishops or special confessors), he has made no move to amend these Directives. United States Conference of Catholic Bishops, *Ethical and Religious Directives for Catholic Health Care Services, Fifth Ed.* (2009), e.g., Directives 45, 47, 52, and 53. Uttley L, Khaikin C. *Growth of Catholic Hospitals and Health Systems*. MergerWatch, 2016.

pleasure, not children.* Making abortion illegal—or using oppressive regulations to make it expensive, time-consuming, and shaming—serves the same goal of earlier laws criminalizing the use of contraceptives: keeping sex and reproduction tied together.

The current surge of opposition to the right to abortion could be interpreted as a sign of how much legal abortion has contributed to changing traditional norms around women's economic and sexual power. According to sociologists Link and Phelan, the interests of stigmatizers become evident when hidden processes don't achieve them. Then stigmatizers work to reinvigorate the system of social control, through "an upswing in direct person-to-person discrimination, an increase in daily indignities, and advocacy for social control policies that might bring things back in line." The public and private roles of American women have changed radically in a relatively short period of time. The emergence of a large group of women who don't need to marry for money or sex is a dramatic change, and allowing women total control over their reproductive destiny may represent "the last straw" in a transition some people still resist.

Conflict is only productive when we're honest about the real reason we're fighting. Unproductive fighting goes in circles, breeding exhaustion and bitterness. Productive fighting might be painful, but the possibility of progress—new understandings and shared solutions—makes those conflicts worth having. This is true in our personal lives (a couple fighting about who should do the dishes won't resolve anything if a suspicion of infidelity is what's really driving their fight), and it's true in our politics. Let's transform our

* Of course women also have sex for reasons other than pleasure or procreation. Sadly, those reasons include situations that range from the serial rape of trafficked women to the coercion and manipulation of abusive relationships to internalized social pressure to perform acts that meet legal standards of consent. My focus on the voluntary acts of the many women who actually want to have sex and enjoy it does not preclude the reality of others.

political bickering into productive fighting by further unpacking the Russian Doll of abortion, and openly discussing how recent social changes are affecting people both practically and emotionally. If the underlying claim driving abortion "health regulations" is that people shouldn't have abortions at all, and if some abortion conflicts are really or largely about issues like gender, sexuality, and religion, it would be more productive to identify our true disagreements and discuss them directly.

III. REALPOLITIK

Abortion can be philosophically challenging, and it also challenges social norms. Realpolitik steers us from philosophy and political theory to practical considerations. What other factors keep the right to abortion embattled? One rarely discussed factor is that many of those who need abortion are among our society's least politically powerful.

Half of all abortion patients (49%) are "poor." In 2014 (the year this data was collected) the federal poverty line was an annual income of $11,670 for a single woman, and $15,730 for a couple or a mother and child. Half of abortion patients fell below this income level.

Another quarter of all abortion patients (26%) are "low income," meaning they have incomes less than two times the poverty level. Together, poor and low-income women account for three out of four abortion patients.

At the beginning of this book I said I didn't have a blueprint for a new conversation. I do, however, have a few suggestions. The first is that we should discuss abortion as an issue of justice.

When a bioethicist analyzes a situation in medicine, justice is one of the four principles that the most common framework in our field, principlism, instructs us to apply. The shocking number of abortion patients who are poor raises serious justice concerns that warrant a new chapter in the American abortion conversation.

We know poverty makes it harder to fend off a whole range of health issues that have both financial and behavioral components, and unintended pregnancy seems no exception. Poor women have *five times* more unintended pregnancies than women with incomes above 200% of the poverty line. Framed as a percentage, in 2011, 60% of all pregnancies of poor women were unintended. For low-income women the rate was 52%. In contrast, for women with incomes above the low-income line the unintended pregnancy rate was 30%.*

Many poor women who decide to end their unintended pregnancy will find that their health insurance doesn't cover ordinary abortion. If her health insurance comes from Medicaid, she'll find the Hyde Amendment limits the federal Medicaid program to coverage only in cases of rape, incest, or life-threatening (but not health-threatening) pregnancy, and the majority of state Medicaid programs have adopted the same restrictions. If she is insured through her job or insurance she bought herself, her private insurance also might not cover ordinary abortion. (Some insurance plans choose not to cover abortion, and others are legally prohibited from doing so. For example, as of 2016, eleven states restrict abortion coverage in private plans.) This is insurance discrimination. The consequence of this insurance discrimination is that a poor woman who can't pay out of pocket could be denied her constitutional right to determine whether and when to give birth to a child.

Or she'll try to find the money to pay out of pocket. (As discussed earlier, if she lives in a state with restrictions or few clinics, in addition

* Discussion of disparities in unintended pregnancy, abortion, and childbearing says nothing about how many children a woman who is poor "should" have. It's an acknowledgment that pregnancies women define as unwanted are something people in all income brackets would prefer to avoid.

to the procedure costs she has to raise additional money to overcome other obstacles.) That takes time, pushing her abortion to later gestational ages. Delay is not good for her, because the risks abortion does have rise as pregnancy advances. And if you, as her neighbor, are more troubled by later abortions than earlier ones, her insurance plan's lack of abortion coverage harms you too.

However, despite the fact poor women are half of abortion patients, these women are *less* likely to terminate an unintended pregnancy than higher-income women. For women living under the poverty line, 38% of unintended pregnancies end in abortion, compared with 48% of unintended pregnancies in women with incomes over 200% of the poverty line. The high rate of unintended pregnancy in this group means that in addition to a higher abortion rate (the number of abortions for every 1,000 women), poor and low-income women also have a higher rate of carrying unintended pregnancies to term than women with higher incomes. In 2011, women below the poverty line delivered 60 unintended pregnancies per 1,000 women, versus 9 per 1,000 for women over 200% of the poverty line.

The fact that half of abortion patients live below the poverty level should give us pause. Considering abortion as a class issue makes anti-abortion policies look like a battle of ideas largely enacted on the bodies of the poor. This is not to say poor women are passive victims lacking agency, it's to say the politically powerful people driving abortion regulation are not usually poor women.

Realpolitik highlights another problem with abortion politics. The competing ideas explored in Chapters 4 and 5 are fascinating. When they're mixed with politics, those ideas are transformed into a legal battle that's become disgraceful.

First, it's deceitful. By definition, a Trojan Horse statute uses false premises to accomplish its goal. For example, as suggested in Chapter 5, twenty-week abortion bans premised on a fetus's capacity to feel pain are a legislative lie. I don't believe the people who pass these laws actually believe fetuses have the capacity to feel pain at twenty weeks. More disturbingly, I don't think they care if what they're saying is true.

The Texas "health and safety" law discussed at the beginning of this chapter is another an example of legislative bad faith. The *Whole Woman's Health* opinion recounts that when the Texas Solicitor General was "directly asked at oral argument whether Texas knew of a single instance in which the new requirement [of admitting privileges] would have helped even one woman obtain better treatment, Texas admitted that there was no evidence in the record of such a case." And the second new requirement? "The upshot is that this record evidence [of ASC standards adding no improvement in patient safety], along with the absence of any evidence to the contrary, provides ample support for the District Court's conclusion" to strike the law as unconstitutional.

Not one case of harm Texas could claim it was trying to prevent from happening again, and no credible evidence the new ASC requirement would improve patient safety. How did Texans who oppose abortion sink so low? You rarely see a sentence like this in a Supreme Court opinion, but this is how the Court interpreted Texas's position: "[I]n the face of no threat to women's health, Texas seeks to force women to travel long distances to get abortions in crammed-to-capacity super facilities. ... [T]hese effects would be harmful to, not supportive of, women's health."

Texas taxpayers should be furious to have financed this circus, including Texans who oppose abortion. Public resources wasted on costly litigation of unconstitutional statutes is money that could have made a real impact preventing abortion through contraceptive access, improving the lives of existing children living in poverty, and so many other "pro-life" causes.

Deceptive diversions from the real issue—whether and when it is morally acceptable to kill an embryo or fetus—preclude us from the kind of productive disagreement that could advance the American abortion conversation. The Trojan Horse trend abuses the trust and wastes the time of well-intentioned people trying to understand the issues. It makes abortion politics and litigation feel like a game in which no one says what they really mean, and that leads many reasonable people to drop out of the abortion discussion in frustration.

Trojan Horse abortion laws are also disrespectful. Imagine if your state legislature was still passing laws requiring segregated public schools forty-five years after *Brown v. Board of Education* ruled "separate but equal" was unconstitutional. That would have felt like an ugly waste of time, wouldn't it? Yet that's what states passing heartbeat bans or twenty-week abortion bans are doing forty-five years after *Roe v. Wade* ruled that banning abortion before viability is unconstitutional. Why? I think disrespect for women is an important part of the equation. A Supreme Court ruling empowering women is not considered a *legitimate* ruling. Not even when it's forty-five years old, not even when the Supreme Court explicitly affirms it nineteen years later in *Casey* in response to your challenges. A ruling that says women have a constitutional right to control their bodies? That can't be a *real* constitutional right. That's still unsettled law. Keep swinging.

So far I've been referring to Trojan Horse abortion laws that are unconstitutional. A second group of these laws is permitted by the Constitution, because the Court adopted the "undue burden" standard in the 1992 case affirming *Roe*. The *Casey* Court explained that when "a state regulation has the purpose or effect of placing a substantial obstacle in the path of a woman seeking an abortion of a nonviable fetus," this is an unacceptable ("undue") burden on the abortion right. As mentioned earlier, the *Casey* Court found one state restriction was an undue burden (spousal notification) and four were not: a twenty-four-hour waiting period, an "informed consent" requirement, parental consent with judicial bypass, and a record-keeping requirement. That's why laws like the "informed consent" and waiting period examples I considered in the discussion of structural stigma aren't usually found to violate the Constitution.

However, just because something is legal doesn't mean it's ethical. This book's discussion of abortion ethics is premised on that fact, and the same analysis should be applied to this group of Trojan Horse abortion laws. *Casey* makes them legal. And they are unethical. As explained in the analysis of clinic blockades, these laws are the codification of assault.

The Trojan Horse trend uses the latitude granted in *Casey* to try to coerce women into having children they do not want. After failing to convince the courts that the Constitution allows states to make abortion illegal, and failing to persuade the approximately one million women (and many of their partners) who request the procedure every year that abortion is immoral, abortion opponents are trying to make abortion unavailable. These laws try to do by force, trick, or trap what fetal rights advocates haven't been able to do by persuasion. Trojan Horse abortion laws are a formalized, privatized way of bullying neighbors who disagree with you, a form of abuse that can't be captured on the nightly news the way clinic assaults were broadcast. Abortion regulation has become a way to knock women around for sport without consequence for those who do it.

The Trojan Horse trend has gone too far. People who believe abortion is wrong, and even people who believe abortion should be illegal, should oppose Trojan Horse abortion laws for the same reasons moderates withdrew their support for the clinic terrorism of the 1980s and early 1990s. It is unethical to attempt to force, badger, cajole, or shame a woman into allowing a pregnancy she never intended to create to result in a child for whom she'll be forever responsible. A physician who did that would be in grave violation of the ethical principle of informed decisionmaking. A legislator or voter who does it also violates this principle. Stop passing these laws.

The conversation we need today is less about abortion, and more about what abortion is doing to us. Forty-five years of abortion wars should propel us to a larger conversation about what kind of country we want to be. A pluralistic country in which robust debates about right and wrong and impassioned efforts to persuade one's neighbors are welcome? Or a country in which the government can force (or forbid) childbearing?

The country we are now is not one of compromise or acceptable accord. States have cast a regulatory net over abortion patients and providers to burden, delay, and shame them. These laws try to come between women and their doctors, women and men they love, women and the children they're already raising, women and their religion, women and their conscience. Abortion is a matter of the heart. The Constitution prohibits the government from imposing one religion's view of ethics on everyone through law, and there are sensible secular ethics arguments for and against abortion. That's why the era of federal and state governments passing morality laws on abortion should end.

What kind of country do we want to be? I vote for pluralism.

The abortion debate often seems to boil down to a debate about vulnerability: Who or what is more in need of protection, fetuses or women? For me, the vulnerable thing in need of protection is pluralism—the idea that Americans who vigorously disagree about gender, family, sex, religion, and endless other topics can all flourish in the same country.

I'm not asking you to like abortion. I'm asking you to like pluralism. I'm asking you to acknowledge that your feeling, opinion, belief, or conviction about the moral status of embryos and fetuses cannot be proven to the level required to force it on others through force of law. In the United States, we can't force a neighbor to end a pregnancy we don't think she should continue, and we can't force a neighbor to continue a pregnancy we don't think she should end.

I'm asking for a new public abortion conversation, one characterized by sincerity of content and civility of tone. I'm asking for respect and compassion for neighbors who disagree. Abortion has been hard, and we all need to rise up and be our best selves to move forward. Before we debate the next set of regulations, we have some conceptual questions to answer. Yes, we disagree about abortion. But what should we make of that fact? What should we do about it? Abortion's legality causes some Americans anguish. What price may the anguished extract from those who aren't? What exactly, if anything, do a patient and a doctor who are not pained by abortion owe a neighbor who is? And what, beyond legality, is owed to them?

I am asking opponents to oppose abortion with integrity. Philosophically, opposing with integrity might mean working to change hearts and minds so women and couples will come to agree with your view and they won't *want* to end accidental pregnancies. (Ideally, persuading people to see things your way before they are pregnant.) Practically, opposing with integrity might mean working to reduce the abortion rate in ways that empower women to define their own futures, such as working to insure that those who don't want to be pregnant have access to the medical resources they need to prevent it, and working to insure that those who want to have children have the social and economic support that make this possible. (As mentioned earlier, 73% of women list the inability to afford another child as one reason they are having an abortion, and 23% list it as the most important reason.) Politically, opposing with integrity means accepting the rulings of *Roe* and *Casey*. Respect for pluralism might lead one to focus on lowering the abortion rate in ways like those named above. (As a wonderful pro-life doctor I work with says, he doesn't want abortion to be illegal, he wants it to be unnecessary.) Alternatively, some honest abolitionists might feel compelled to campaign for a constitutional amendment that would clearly contradict *Roe* and *Casey* by granting embryos and fetuses constitutional rights superior to women's constitutional rights.

I am asking supporters to support abortion with courage. Many people aspire to appear apolitical on abortion. That usually means staying quiet about it, even in relevant professions like medicine and academia. The common meaning of "apolitical," not involved or interested in politics, isn't quite right; they might have strong opinions on abortion policy. It's usually the second meaning, an aversion to politics, that's relevant. They're repulsed by the vitriol of abortion politics, which has made talking about abortion at all feel unseemly or even dangerous. So they stay quiet, to avoid being seen as "taking a side."

The problem is, whether you intend it or not, and whether you like it or not, when the constitutional right to self-determination is being denied, burdened, or stigmatized, silence *is* "taking a side." In this polarized public debate, silence speaks—a tacit statement that it's okay to let reproductive rights slip away. Silence on abortion is also an exercise of privilege. Ignoring the needs of millions of poor people, young people, and women is not "apolitical." (Nor is ignoring the needs of embryos and fetuses, if that's where you think vulnerability lies.)

Even if "apolitical" were the goal, that's not synonymous with "silent." An ordinary level of open support for other common, legal medical procedures isn't considered political. (And in my field, silence in other controversial areas of medicine—from genetics to childhood vaccinations to who is first in line for organ transplant—wouldn't be apolitical, it'd be negligent.) Abortion is a constitutional right that somewhere between a third and a quarter of American women exercise at some point in their lives. Silence on this topic isn't apolitical, it's abandonment.

Abortion is treated as if it's different from the rest of health care. There are ways in which abortion *is* different. Ironically, the segregation produced by its political framing has become an important actual difference. The idea that "staying out of abortion" is the apolitical choice is a product of stigma.

Instead of apolitical, let's aspire to be nonpartisan. "Partisan" means prejudiced, discriminatory, or one-sided. Positions are partisan when they are preordained, and people are partisan when they're unable to integrate new information or unwilling to consider changing their mind. The topic of abortion isn't inherently partisan, although the way it's approached often is. Let's work to make disagreement civil and fruitful, instead of assuming disagreement will be ugly and unproductive. Instead of suppressing conflict, let's shepherd it to a softer space, and wrestle with it in good faith.

Let's take the energy and goodwill we save by dialing down the public vitriol and gamesmanship, and invest it into more robust private conversations about abortion. Let's move thoughtful discussion of abortion ethics and abortion experience into the realm of normal conversation between students eating pizza in the dorm, people in romantic relationships in which an unintended pregnancy could happen, parents and teenagers, doctors and patients, friends at book club, and your next dinner party. Start with people you know and like, and risk being vulnerable with them. I don't want a culture of life, and I don't want a culture of abortion. I want a culture of permission. Permission to share your experiences, permission to keep things private, permission to articulate your values, permission to disagree, permission to feel uncertain and unsettled. Permission to step up and do the hard thing that's the right thing, whether for you that's having a baby or having an abortion. Permission to forgive and move on.

So tell people you trust what the abortion you participated in was like for you, or tell them how happy you are that you or a loved one didn't end that accidental pregnancy, or tell them what you think or hope you might do if you're ever in that situation, or tell them what you hope other people will do and why.

One hundred and thirteen women in the legal profession told the Supreme Court that they'd had abortions. Professor Sylvia Law was among those who "came out" in an amicus brief submitted in the *Whole Woman's Health* litigation, signing their names to say that although their abortion stories were different, they were "united in their strongly-held belief that they would not have been able to achieve the personal or professional successes they have achieved were it not for their ability to obtain safe and legal abortions."

They also overcame an obstacle to abortion storytelling. Their abortion wasn't just an event that happened in the past, it was both the beginning of the story of the rest of their lives, and the end of an alternate story they didn't want to be part of.

> *I am the daughter of a teenage mother who is the daughter of a teenage mother. I had an abortion when I was 16 years old and living in rural Oregon. I believe that access to safe, legal abortion broke the familial cycle of teenage parenthood and allowed me to not only escape a very unhealthy, emotionally abusive teenage relationship but to graduate from an elite college, work for one of the nation's most storied civil rights organizations, and go on to graduate from the University of Michigan Law School.*

> *I had an abortion at age 35, when I had an unplanned pregnancy with a man who had become emotionally abusive. … I was firm in my belief that my happiness and that of any family I would start begins with the stability of my relationship with a partner. … I eventually found that [amazing] man and married him at age 42. We are blessed with two amazing sons. I went on to become the general counsel of an international energy consulting firm … and know that my family and career would not have been as joyful and successful had I not had the option to choose when to start a family.*

> *My abortion made it possible for me to reinhabit my body as an individual. After nine months of pregnancy and a year of breastfeeding, regaining whole possession of my body was essential to my autonomy and mental health. … My abortion also made it possible for me to continue to build my career as a public defender.*

If Hester Prynne lived today, hopefully she and minister Arthur Dimmesdale would benefit from our era's advances in contraception. If they did have an accidental pregnancy, our era's reduced social stigma around illegitimate children would make having a child together a real option. Or perhaps Hester, whether independently or together with Arthur, would decide to have an abortion.

> *I was terrified when I realized I was pregnant—I'm from a conservative immigrant community that would've pilloried me—but access to safe legal abortion changed my life. Instead of living as an outcast trying to scrape out an existence selling my sewing, I was able to leave my hometown and chase my dream of becoming a clothing designer. I'm never happier than when I'm creating. Except when I'm with Arthur. It took him a few years to get up the guts to follow me, but now he loves working at an impoverished parish famous for its parenting classes, and playing with our daughters Hope, Grace, and Connie. Twenty years later, I'm still irritated by the way he cuts his toenails on the couch, still delighted by the way he turns up the kitchen radio and spins me while we cook, and still bound to him through our shared love of God, our kids, our work, and the kind of sex that's worth getting banished for. Has the life I've lived been perfect? Far from it. But for better and worse, it's been mine.*

Epilogue

I was honored to be invited to talk with hundreds of women's health care providers from across Latin America. I shared ideas from this book, then went to bed giddy, but not because of the conference. The second I woke I lunged for the drugstore pregnancy test I'd brought, peed on a stick, and cried in a hotel bathroom. The irony was not lost on me: millions of women accidentally get pregnant every year, and I'm here lecturing about their option to end it. I'm very intentionally trying to get pregnant, and after lots and lots of work, it's still not happening.

When I finally did get pregnant, my husband and I were ecstatic. Ten weeks later, we got bad news.

Professors don't usually write about their personal lives. In medicine that raises interesting questions, since everyone's private life interacts with that field in one way or another. Is the fact an oncologist had cancer herself relevant in her oncology research articles? Is the painful death of a bioethicist's mother relevant to his writing on the ethics of physician-assisted dying? Whether professors shifting their narrative stance from analyst to subject enriches or undermines their intellectual analysis is a case-by-case question. But intimate experience isn't considered a "conflict of interest" that *requires* disclosure. People writing about pediatrics don't need to drop a footnote disclosing whether they've had children, and people writing about abortion have no obligation to share whether they have been part of one or not.

Yet privacy and integrity are in tension for me here. "Shout Your Abortion" is a social media campaign that invites women to videotape themselves telling their abortion stories for viewing on YouTube. I applaud women who donate personal narratives for public discussion, but as a student once put it, "I don't want to 'shout my abortion.' I just want to be able to mention it when it's relevant."

That's exactly how I feel. So why hold myself to a different standard? Because deep in the process of writing a book about one of the most contentious topics in America, I unexpectedly found myself facing the procedure I was writing about. I'd prefer to not discuss my experience publicly—it's no one else's business, and I hate the idea of hate mail. And what I've advocated in this book is candid private conversation, so I don't think it would be hypocritical of me to not publicly expose this part of my private life. Then I picture all the doctors, nurses, and clinic managers I met while working on this book who collectively care for millions of silent women at such personal risk to themselves, and medical privacy seems a privilege that costs them too much. I picture the doctor I met the day I needed help, and gratitude for her care obligates me to leave my comfort zone. I picture the women who shared their stories with me for publication, and solidarity requires me to join them. I am not special. And I am not ashamed.

This story involves my husband's privacy too. We created that pregnancy together, and we made our decision and took our action to end it together. "Consent" is insufficient for intimates—I share our story here only because he gave me his full endorsement for doing so, for which I am incredibly grateful.

So I'll tell you that I was pregnant, and we got bad news, and we had a decision to make. I choose not to share our diagnosis because I want to retain at least that amount of privacy. I'm comforted by the possibility this omission might actually make it a better story to think with. If it was a severe physical disability that had no impact on cognition, what would you think of me? What if it was a severe mental disability with no impact on the rest of the body? Moderate impairment of both physical and cognitive function? If death was inevitable hours after the umbilical cord was cut at delivery, would you think ours such an obvious, sympathetic choice that it was not even a "real abortion"? What if it were Down syndrome (trisomy 21—three copies of the 21st chromosome), which can turn out to be severe, moderate or mild, but genetic testing can't say which version it will be? What if it were trisomy 13 or trisomy 18, which typically result in multiple organ defects, severe developmental delays, and very short lifespans? What if I had changed my mind, and I just plain didn't want to have a baby? Is there a difference between what you could approve for yourself, and what you can allow for someone else? Are there reasons for my action that would lead you to decide you and I couldn't be friends?

Our diagnosis came at twelve weeks LMP (the way pregnancy is calculated, that's ten weeks after conception) and confirming it took two more weeks of testing, which means I ended the pregnancy in the second trimester, around fourteen weeks LMP. Some would call this a "late" abortion, but we did it as early as we could. A sonogram can't reveal anatomical problems like a fatal absence of kidneys, or devastating lack of brain growth, before all the body parts are supposed to be in place, and that happens around the turn from the first to second trimester. (Sadly, sometimes an organ defect such as a malformed heart can be *seen* at twelve weeks, but doctors can't tell if it's fatal or fixable until the organ grows to the size it reaches toward the end of the second trimester.) This screening also includes genetic testing, which identifies missing or extra pieces of fetal DNA that will lead to body or brain differences of varying severity and probability.

Before we tried to get pregnant, my husband and I discussed the limits of our parenting capacities. We felt moral authority to draw a line, the diagnosis fell on the other side of our line, and living with the reality of the diagnosis did not change our earlier decision. It sounds cold when I write it, but it was not. It was filled with tears, but not with doubts. I understood our limits as a negative commentary on us, not on the worth of our fetus or any person with a disability.* Does that mean I'd cease to parent the child I have now if the results of an accident or disease put him on the other side of that line? Of course not—I would devote everything I have to give him the best life possible. That is the unspoken pledge I made when I chose to have a baby. It is not the pledge I made when I got pregnant.

So I called the hospital that made the diagnosis to see what our options were while we waited for follow-up testing. The woman who scheduled abortions was incredibly nice. Along with the medical and practical details, she reviewed our insurance and said we'd have a 20% copay. It was only at the end of the call that I thought to ask how much the procedure cost—20% of what? "$20,000 or more." I was floored. I wouldn't ordinarily ask the cost of a medical procedure covered by insurance, but about ten years ago I'd heard that first-trimester abortions in a hospital could be three to four times more expensive than in clinics. But $20,000? I asked if other private clinics in town did second-trimester procedures, and she said yes.

"Does it cost less there?"

"It does."

"Do you have any sense of how much they charge?"

"At Planned Parenthood it's like $720."

"For the same procedure???"

"Yes, so that's where we refer people who are paying out of pocket. But sometimes people with insurance prefer to come here."

* I'm influenced by the compelling disability rights critiques of abortion for "fetal indications," and saddened by the gap between the social message one does or does not intend, and the message that might reasonably be received.

"Why?" I asked, expecting a speech about quality.

"Because they don't want to deal with protesters. Or they don't want to go to an abortion clinic."

"An abortion clinic? But it's the same procedure."

"Not really. Yours isn't elective. You didn't have a choice."

False. She was trying to be kind, telling me I was having a Nice Lady Abortion—that as a woman with a wanted pregnancy and a medical problem I was different from women who go to "abortion clinics." But I'm not. Of course I had a choice—we're always making choices. Some choices are just more common, or more comprehensible to others. "Extraordinary abortion" can be comfortably fit into the disease and injury paradigm of medical care, but our decision that we did not want to parent a child with this particular diagnosis seems no better or worse to me than a couple with three children deciding they can't take on a fourth, or a woman deciding she'd rather not be a single parent. All are questions of time, resources, values, and your vision for your own life and family.

But a prestigious hospital versus a clinic? That isn't the kind of decision you want to base on money if you can afford otherwise. I was lucky to be able to pose this question to a wonderful doctor who specializes in second-trimester abortions, and who worked in all the local clinics, as well as the hospital I was considering, during her training. Would the hospital and the clinic provide comparable care? No, she said—the clinic is better. Their method takes three to six hours. The hospital's method takes two visits over two days, and the hospital insists on doing second-trimester procedures in an operating room, so you pay full operating room and anesthesia costs, which she felt were unnecessary. She said the clinic's method "would be my choice. You will be in good hands."

The receptionist at the clinic was not as put-together as the hospital scheduler. "No fingernail or toenail polish, no food or drink eight hours before, bring two maxi-pads." BYOMP? That felt bizarrely cut-rate. (Yes, hospitals provide maxi-pads, but they probably charge $20 each, I told myself. BYOMP. Check.) I have to have someone drive me there and drive me home, and they have to stay the whole time. THEY HAVE TO STAY THE WHOLE TIME. The third time she said it, I said, "Yes, my husband will be there." "Ohhh!" her voice went up an approving octave. She said I'd get birth control counseling before the procedure, then when I'm in the recovery room I'd get the birth control method I selected. I kept my mouth shut—she probably doesn't get many patients with fertility challenges and wanted pregnancies.

My state doesn't have a mandated waiting period, but the structure of medical care provided one anyway. One thing the hospital and the clinic have in common is that both do abortions only two days a week. The way prenatal testing works added more time. After our screening test brought bad news, we had to wait four days until we could do the more precise test. Two days later we got preliminary results from this second test (confirming the diagnosis with 99.5% accuracy). Based on the clinic's "abortion days," we could've done it a few days after that, but I've read too many Greek tragedies to do it before the 100% confirmation came in. Wanting that last confirmation required us to wait another seven to ten days, but I very much wanted to be in that 0.5%. So we booked the procedure for seven days later, hoping to beat the odds and adjusting to what was 99.5% likely. The days between knowing what we were going to do and doing it were excruciating. Sadly, that happens to be a week a fetus almost doubles in size. I could feel my belly start to pop, and I wanted to crawl out of my skin. No baby, no you gorgeous thing, no. The 100% confirmation came in seven days later, the afternoon before our appointment. Yes, we are doing this.

Usually I'd wear sweatpants to a medical procedure, but the thought of walking through a picket line drives me to dress up. I put on a stretchy long skirt, a nice top, and a cardigan. I put on makeup and do my hair. The receptionist said no jewelry, but it feels important to me to wear my wedding ring and earrings. I want protesters to see my put-together self; that's who I want and need to be to brave a line of angry strangers on my way to get medical care I'm sad to need and have a constitutional right to receive. My husband comes downstairs wearing jeans and a softball t-shirt. "Humor me and put on a nicer shirt?" He cocks his head as if about to ask why, then wordlessly jogs up the stairs to change.

We arrive 30 minutes early so we'll have time to assess the best way to enter and to steel ourselves for facing a crowd. We circle the block, and there's not a single protester outside. This has been true the few other times I've passed this clinic, but what the hospital scheduler said spooked me and I didn't know if today would be different. It isn't. We park the car, sit, and begin laughing at our nice outfits and free time.

"See!" I say to my husband. "Ordinary abortion! They don't all have protesters."

"Yeah, I didn't see any reference to them on Yelp."

"You Yelped our abortion clinic?"

Past a grim security measure, the interior of the clinic is sunny and antiseptic. With its bright paint, fake maple flooring, and green Formica counters, its only difference from other medical offices is the surfeit of tattoos on the nursing staff. I'm asked how I'll pay and feel the impulse to keep this visit separate from the rest of my bureaucratically surveilled life by paying out of pocket. But a study I read finding that a large number of women with private insurance still choose to pay for their abortion themselves struck me as a sad, expensive expression of abortion stigma, and remembering that keeps me on track. Pulling out my insurance card suddenly feels like a political statement. Why else do we pay all those premiums?

I meet with the clinic's counselor. She asks me about my feelings, decisionmaking process, and social support, and it's all well and good but I can't help staring at a wicker breadbasket on her desk filled with medical instruments and plastic food. Like the gun introduced in Act One, I become fixated on when and how the breadbasket will go off. Finally she shows me the instruments they'll use in the procedure. Then she holds up a plastic egg to say that even after the pregnancy is removed, "it's normal to have blood clots of this size." She holds up a plastic lemon . . . and memory fails me here, were lemon clots the bad ones? Or was that the dinner roll?

I'm given two pills that will soften my cervix so it can be dilated. I'm told to put them between my cheek and gum until they dissolve, then wait two hours. The form says side effects can include vomiting, diarrhea, cramping, and bleeding, but thankfully I just have mild cramping. I pull my feet up into my stretchy skirt, cuddle my husband across our plastic chairs to stay warm, and pull out my book to pass the time. But I can't concentrate on *The Goldfinch* because a large TV is blaring *The View* at unholy volumes, and the only magazines available seem to be *Runner's World* and *Ladies' Home Journal*. If this is the media content of Feminazi headquarters, Rush Limbaugh needn't be so concerned. The most ordinary not-ordinary doctor's visit ever.

Two hours is a long time to look around a waiting room. It was pretty crowded—maybe sixty people that day? About thirty pairs of friends, lovers, mothers and daughters, and women who looked like sisters, all in their own private world keeping to themselves. When I told my sister about it later she was surprised by the lack of privacy ("What if you saw someone you knew?"), but from that perspective it was the same as any other specialist's office—whether it's allergies or obstetrics, you know what everyone else in the waiting room is there for. It reminded me of my grandmother's cataracts. She and my father used to joke about going to the "eye factory," a specialty clinic packed with people waiting to efficiently go through the same minor surgery. They had no complaint with the medical quality and said the doctors were nice, but I think it still felt like a mill to them, impersonal eye care that wasn't integrated with the rest of her health care. I once spoke with a woman who seemed to feel similarly about her abortion clinic experience; she said sitting with everyone else made her uncomfortable and she was upset she couldn't do it with her own ob/gyn. I didn't mind, it just reminded me that a lot of people do this. And I knew that whether it's cataract surgery, pregnancy termination, or hernia repair, the upside of focusing on one procedure in one location is often higher-quality medical care at lower cost. So I retreat back to the cocoon of my skirt and my husband's arm, and try to focus on my book.

I go back for the procedure, and after some conversation with a friendly ob/gyn, anesthesiologist, and nurse, the next thing I know I'm in a recovery room full of pink vinyl recliners containing patients connected to IV poles. The doctor comes to tell me I bled "more than you should" in the procedure, so they're going to monitor me here longer than usual. A nurse walks me to the bathroom and the relevance of the plastic egg tutorial becomes vivid. I'm woozy and jealous of the women I overhear reporting their cramps are "0" on the 1–10 scale, then after fifteen minutes in the recliner, report their bleeding is light to nonexistent. Those women get water and a little packet of Goldfish crackers while their "guests" come to the door to take them home. I become obsessed with wanting those dumb crackers, but the blood is still coming and I can't eat or drink in case they have to do something else to stop the bleeding. So I recline for almost two hours until the bleeding resolves and they confirm my vitals and hemoglobin are stable.

As I said earlier in this book, abortion is a very safe procedure. But like all medical procedures, part of its safety record depends on the legality that allows it to be done by professionals in medical settings. It turns out I'm a bleeder—after delivering my baby I hemorrhaged horribly (way more). If abortion had been illegal, and this was a clandestine abortion in some hidden apartment, my surprise bleeding could've been life-threatening. Instead, proper medical management meant it only cost me an extra two hours of lusting for crackers and watching dumb products float by on QVC TV.

We got home late Wednesday afternoon, and I slept from 7:00 p.m. to 11:30 a.m. Thursday and Friday I stayed home to rest and putter. By Sunday I felt significantly better, both physically and emotionally. The doctor who advised me to go to the clinic instead of the hospital gave me a second piece of good advice: "Mourn your loss, and celebrate the life you nurtured for three months." So Sunday afternoon I sobbed as I taped our most recent sonogram picture in my journal, and wrote him/her/it a letter explaining why we did what we did and saying goodbye.

Monday night we had dinner with a kind friend. He asked how I was doing. Then he asked, with genuine curiosity and openness, if having an abortion made me feel any differently about the topic of my book. I was struck by how nice it was to be asked to talk about my abortion, as if it's a normal thing people are allowed to talk about over dinner. And I've continued to ponder his question.

My experience affirmed my belief that hearing a range of stories can help us locate our own when it's our turn. Having heard other women's abortion experiences and opinions helped me contextualize my own emotions and thinking. Doing this work also emboldened me to reach out for support. We told quite a few sympathetic friends and family we were ending a pregnancy, more than the number who knew we were pregnant in the first place. That turned out to be a huge advantage in our recovery, because people called, texted, and emailed in the days afterward, and their love and concern buoyed us. I was surprised and moved that two couples sent flowers. I called to thank one, and the spouse who answered the phone stammered apologetically. "Was that the right thing to do? Because you suffered a loss. Not a death ... unless you feel like it's a death, then absolutely it's a death. But we didn't know. Because you send flowers when someone's sick, so either way, we just—I hope that was okay." (More than okay. Affirming and wonderful.) I know not every woman will get this response; much of it probably stemmed from the fact this began as a wanted pregnancy. Yet it struck me that another cost of abortion secrecy is the lost opportunity for unexpected empathy.

Actually it's the pregnancy I carried to term that intensified my views on abortion most. As billions have experienced, it is the most concrete demonstration of potentiality possible—a single cell turned into my beloved boy. Knowing who my son is today, it's easy to project his personhood backward into the womb. I don't think that blastocyst, or embryo, or fetus was my son. But of course they became him—without them, there is no him. No pro-life argument will convince me an embryo is a person. And no pro-choice position will make me forget that an embryo a woman continues to nurture will become one.

But it's the nurturance we forget, and what being pregnant reminded me to respect. At one prenatal visit the midwife said I should take calcium supplements. I responded like a smug know-it-all: "Because the baby needs it to build bones." She looked at me for a moment, calculating. "The baby takes everything it needs from your body. The calcium is for you." My baby is eating my bones? I would've endured the calcium-induced constipation for his benefit, but the vision of replenishing his metaphoric nibbles into my bones was further motivating.

Mine was a completely average pregnancy—some have it worse, and some have it better. Reading a journal entry from the first trimester reminded me of what's easy to forget: being pregnant is a part-time job.

> I'm at real week 5.5, LMP week 7.5, and I feel really bad. If I'd never heard of pregnancy, I'd think I had cancer—it feels like something is eating me from the inside; like something in my

> body has fundamentally changed for the worse. I've moved from queasy to nauseous, hours and hours of salivating and feeling like I'm GOING to throw up, which is horrible. And I'm so exhausted—sometimes I can't sleep more than 4 or 5 hours a night, and I'm on pregnant lady time, which means I really want 9–10! Sunday night I wept from misery and frustration and nausea and exhaustion. Poor [husband] thought I was crazy—he was watching TV while I marched up and down the staircase, over and over again, crying the whole time, because being in motion was the only thing that helped the nausea at all. ("There isn't anything I can do?" "No!" Cry-cry-cry, walk-walk-walk.) And my exhausted mush-brain has messed up a hundred things at work. I think of myself as strong, but something no bigger than a grain of rice is kicking my ass. How is that possible? I feel worn down and worthless. I work to reframe—Honeycrisp [our nickname for our tiny friend] and I are on the same team, it's buffeted by hormone storms too, it's not trying to hurt me. But on unsentimental days, my exhausted brain thinks of Honeycrisp as a parasite that's on the brink of violating the cardinal rule of symbiosis—don't kill the host!

In retrospect my journal entries about the difficulties of pregnancy seem "dear" to me. Today I'm focused on my sweet child, and I'd forgotten most of those symptoms until I went back and read what I wrote about them. (An evolutionary amnesia that makes us want to do it again?) But it's good to remember what it was like to feel "occupied," sharing my body with a selfish roommate. Because pregnancy is common, and its outcome is often so joyful, it's easy to forget how much work it is. Pregnancy is profound, intimate, physical labor. I had every advantage—a supportive partner, flexible work hours, good nutrition, health care, a comfortable home, and no other children to care for. And still, it was hard. (Then comes the pain and medical risk of childbirth, and the phenomenal time and emotional investment of parenting.) Mine was a passionately wanted pregnancy, yet physically carrying my beloved still felt like a desperate imposition, an invasion of the body snatchers. If I didn't want the end result of pregnancy, I cannot imagine how horrible it would be to be forced by the government to endure it.

As Justice O'Connor, the first Supreme Court Justice in American history who had experienced pregnancy, explained it in the majority opinion in the 1992 case that affirmed *Roe v. Wade* (*Casey*), "[T]he liberty of the woman is at stake in a sense unique to the human condition, and so, unique to the law. The mother who carries a child to full term is subject to anxieties, to physical constraints, to pain that only she must bear. ... Her suffering is too intimate and personal for the State to insist, without more, upon its own vision of the woman's role... ." An acquaintance said the same thing to me more plainly after having her third baby: "The more children I have, the more pro-choice I get."

The first time I was pregnant I made up a series of little songs I'd sing to my embryo under my breath while I was jogging. They made me happy; they made me feel close to my someday-baby. The second time I was pregnant there was a day I spontaneously began singing one of these little songs on a jog, then quickly stopped, sick to my stomach in a different way. It felt like a gross betrayal—singing this one songs inspired by love for another. I think of my first fetus as something deserving of my respect. Not so much that I didn't have authority to end its life. Enough that I would never sing its songs to another. It took longer with my second pregnancy, to risk loving the creature first nicknamed Honeycrisp, and later Dinosaur Jr. for the way he roiled and kicked like a baby pterodactyl trying to peck its way out of a giant egg. But soon I made up new songs, just for him.

I don't have mixed feelings about my abortion. I do have mixed feelings about writing about my abortion. Some people in my life might be upset to learn I did this, and perhaps they'll think less of me. Some who know and approve of my action might be upset with my choice to acknowledge it in print, perhaps feeling I've publicly tainted them by association. Some who know me professionally are likely to think it a waste of paper—medical researchers might find it distracting, and those steeped in abortion stories might find it banal. Someday my son might want to know more about this, or maybe he'll wish he knew less. Amazingly, complete strangers might feel it's appropriate to tell me I'm a baby killer. Perhaps other strangers will say they have a story they'd like to tell too.

And, here we all are. Let's keep talking.

ACKNOWLEDGMENTS

Like wine, every book like this is a product of the academic terroir in which it grew. The unique interdisciplinary environment created by my Medical Humanities and Bioethics colleagues at Northwestern's Feinberg School of Medicine is the only one in which it could have been written, and I thank everyone in the group for fostering the collegial cross-pollination that made it—and me—what we are. Former Program Director Kathryn Montgomery saw and encouraged the academic inside the lawyer, former Program Director Tod Chambers committed himself to creating space for curiosity-driven scholarship, and both modeled what it means to be ambitious, creative, careful thinkers and committed teachers. I'm grateful to literary scholar Catherine Belling and historian Sarah Rodriguez for their feedback on individual chapters and being wonderful colleagues. Medical anthropologist Megan Crowley-Matoka and clinical ethicist and psychologist Debjani Mukherjee were my marathon medics, and for years of reading and discussing rambling drafts in our writing group I can't thank them enough.

I am also very grateful to Carole Joffe, Ph.D. and Julie Chor, M.D. for reading entire chapters; to Larry Cochard, Ph.D., Stephanie Kukora, M.D., Jim Baker, Ph.D., Lori Gawron, M.D., and Mary Ellen Pavone, M.D., for educating me with feedback on or discussion of specific sections; and to Laura Kessler, J.D., and student Briana Allen at the University of Utah's S.J. Quinney College of Law for helping me learn more about Utah law and the case of J.M.S.

Stanley Henshaw, Ph.D. and Rachel Jones, Ph.D. of the Guttmacher Institute are amazing. They were incredibly generous answering my questions about their data, and for taking the time to make special tabulations when what they'd published didn't answer what I asked.

Three people played a larger role in this book's existence than they know. Dr. Cassing Hammond is the person who invited me to give a plenary lecture at the National Abortion Federation (NAF) after the death of Dr. George Tiller in 2009. I had never heard of this group before, and I have attended its conferences almost every year since. Learning about this medical specialty from those in the trenches has been a tremendous gift. Working as a bioethicist has led me to meet many wonderful doctors, but the commitment this group has to the health and well-being of their patients is unparalleled, and what some of them go through to meet their patients' needs is remarkable. My commitments to medicine, social justice, and law have all been nourished by seeing the research presented at NAF conferences, and I hope more bioethicists will be drawn to working in this area of medical practice in the future.

The others who helped inspire this book are my editor at Oxford University Press, Lucy Randall, and my research assistant, Naomi Scheinerman. I was yapping about these ideas in talks, but the idea of a book was just a flirtatious longing. Then each separately emailed me every several months for what I want to say was years—Lucy saying if I did write a book she wanted to publish it, and Naomi saying if I did she wanted to be my research assistant—and the sustained interest of these two sharp women in their twenties is what made me believe someone besides my mom might read it. (Naomi is a Ph.D. student in political theory at Yale, and she is going to be a great professor. Tip to world: hire her!)

Three anonymous reviewers read sample chapters, and I am indebted to them for their wisdom. Buckets of love to the reviewer who read it again as a whole—his or her investment, intelligence, and insight made this book infinitely better.

When the chips are down, call in the playwrights. At the frantic end Novid Parsi and Shayne Kennedy leapt at my plea for fresh eyes in a hurry and gave me the exact regular-person feedback on the entire manuscript I needed at exactly the right time.

Northwestern has the world's most wonderful students. In 2007 some from the first cohort of our master's program in bioethics and medical humanities read about fetal personhood with me in a tutorial, and years later some read draft chapters from a potentially actual book in the same context. In between I've had the pleasure of discussing several ideas from this book in lectures, and I thank my M.A. students and medical students for all they've taught me.

I am grateful to two eminent institutions, a bioethics research group called the Hastings Center, and an abortion research group in the Obstetrics and Gynecology Department of the University of California, San Francisco called ANSIRH (Advancing New Standards in Reproductive Health). Both granted me two-week stints as a Visiting Scholar to work on this book and present material, and the generous and accomplished scholars in both places advanced my thinking and writing greatly. I also thank the University of Chicago Pritzker School of Medicine, the

University of Utah School of Medicine, Harvard Medical Students for Choice, and Beth Israel Deaconess Medical Center for inviting me to lecture on the ideas I was developing.

I was visibly pregnant during the two weeks I spent at ANSIRH. Almost every one of these abortion researchers also happened to be a parent, and halfway through my visit I realized that every meeting I had to discuss academic aspects of abortion began with supportive inquiries about my pending parenthood, stories of their own, or graphic advice on breastfeeding. Later a woman in this group saw both our names on a conference program, and emailed to offer to babysit my son while I gave my paper if I was bringing him. I have many wonderful colleagues in bioethics, but the level of interest in, and support of, family among people in the field of abortion might surprise outsiders. Abortion providers have been uniquely family-friendly as well. They are typically obstetricians and family medicine doctors who chose these fields to support women and families, and the majority of professionals in abortion care are women themselves. As a result, their conferences contain more babies in slings and breastfeeding during presentations, and more demands to see my own baby pictures, than I've experienced anywhere else. Were I to take a hidden video of abortion providers and researchers to post on the internet, it would reveal that behind closed doors, they are a wild pack of baby lovers.

My biggest debt is to my husband. His sustained cheerleading, cooking, and weekend child care is the only reason I was able to move this project out of the endless purgatory of Almost Done. Nobody gets a book out the door without a partner who understands how much it means to them, and I thank my lucky stars every day that my love is also such a wonderful father and teammate.

And finally, I want to offer my heartfelt thanks to everyone who shared their stories with me, whether they appear in this book or not. Your candor has made my world richer, and your generosity in allowing others to engage with your experiences is inspiring.

When this book neared completion, my work as an ethicist led groups to nominate and elect me to two new volunteer positions. First I was asked to join the Board of Directors for NAF and became chair of that board's Ethics Committee. NAF is the professional association of abortion providers in North America—its members care for more than half the women who choose to have abortions in the United States and Canada every year—and it contributes to abortion safety through quality improvement programs, standards of care, protocols, and accredited continuing medical education. (The *New York Times Magazine* referred to NAF as a "mini-AMA," noting that "[abortion] is the only field in medicine to have one or need one.") I've also become a member of the Planned Parenthood Federation of America's National Medical Committee, and that Committee's Bioethics Advisor, and I look forward to going to my first meeting later this year. I accepted these new roles so I can continue learning about this area of health care, and to contribute to preserving its quality and ethical standards.

When the book was just about finished I decided to dust off my bar card. In 2017, I accepted a second job as Senior Counsel at the American Civil Liberties Union of Illinois's Women's and Reproductive Rights Project. I thank them inviting me spend part of each week putting my ethics analysis into action, for accommodating my kooky professor schedule, and the opportunity to learn from the incomparable Lorie Chaiten and an entire office of inspiring advocates. The rest of each week I remain a professor at Northwestern's Feinberg School of Medicine, where I continue my work in bioethics scholarship and teaching our fabulous students.

A NOTE ON METHODS

I never set out to do research on abortion stories. I had no hypothesis. I did not recruit interview subjects, or seek a particular number, or a representative sample to interview. The stories in this book are an organic part of the personal journey it reflects—spend enough years telling people at conferences and cookouts you're writing a book about abortion, and you will be amazed at how many spontaneously share their own experiences. (Or silently point to themselves with a raised eyebrow or nod that says "I had one of those.") When people volunteered stories in informal settings, or in the few instances in which I had learned something through a personal or professional conversation before I began this project, I went back and asked those individuals permission to speak with them for quotation in this book. Institutional Review Board (IRB) approval was not required for these conversations because they do not fit the IRB definition of "research": a systematic investigation (a prospective plan that collects data to answer a question) designed to develop or contribute to generalizable knowledge. The stories in this book are offered only as illustrations and anecdotes that are good to think with.

NOTES

Introduction

PAGE 1: (Foundling Wheel) A student who visited San Spirito Hospital years later told me a plaque explaining the Foundling Wheel has been added to the building. My (now lost) guidebook claimed Pope Innocent had it installed after he dreamed the Tiber River was overflowing with dead babies. Historian John Boswell reproduces three illustrations from a 15th-century manuscript, which describes the founding of the Hospital of the Holy Spirit in Rome in the late 12th century, depicting women throwing their babies into the Tiber, fishermen pulling them out, and fishermen bringing these dead bodies to the Pope. (268–270) Boswell says the story told in these paintings "is neither inherently unlikely nor verifiable." (416) My guidebook's assertion of 1198, the beginning of Pope Innocent's reign, might have been early—but according to Boswell, "Santo Spirito in Rome was clearly caring for foundlings by the fourteenth century." (415) Infanticide is different from abandonment, in which an infant is left in a place where it might be rescued or it might die, but centuries ago the rates of both appear to be shockingly high. Records from Florence in the first half of the 15th century suggest approximately half of abandonments were a result of social catastrophe (famine, poverty, war) or personal difficulty, about half were illegitimate, and about a third had slave mothers and unidentified fathers, "presumably owners or other free members of the household." (419–420) Sadly, after abandonment foundlings faced high rates of death from infectious disease, and high odds of being "adopted" as unpaid household labor. (421) The practice of abandonment continued far beyond Pope Innocent's time—in Toulouse in the eighteenth century the rate of *known* abandonment was one in four children (in poor quarters it was around 40%, in rich parishes around 15%). In Lyons between 1750 and 1789, approximately one-third of babies were abandoned, and in Paris during the same period children known to have been abandoned account for between 20% and 30% of the registered births. (15) "[F]ragmentary evidence suggests very similar urban abandonment rates ranging from 15 to 30 percent of registered births." (16) John Boswell, *The Kindness of Strangers: The Abandonment of Children in Western Europe from Late Antiquity to the Renaissance* (University of Chicago Press, 1988).

PAGE 2: (unsafe abortion) Carole Joffe, "Abortion in historical perspective." In: Maureen Paul, E. Steven Lichtenberg, Lynn Borgatta, David A. Grimes, and Philip G. Stubblefield, eds. *A Clinician's Guide to Medical and Surgical Abortion* (Churchill Livingstone, 1999), 3–10.

PAGE 2: (safe illegal abortion) Laura Kaplan, *The Story of Jane: The Legendary Underground Feminist Abortion Service* (University of Chicago Press, 1995).

PAGE 2: (abortion mortality compared to dental procedure) Raymond EG, Grossman D, Weaver MA, Toti S, Winikoff B. Mortality of induced abortion, other outpatient surgical procedures and common activities in the United States. *Contraception.* 2014;90:476–479.

PAGE 3: My thanks to Sidney Callahan for this framing: "The difference is that abortion for some is late contraception, and for others, infanticide." She and her husband edited a book of pro-choice and pro-life women's perspectives that still resonates today. Sidney Callahan and Daniel Callahan, eds. *Abortion: Understanding Differences* (Plenum Press, 1984), 291.

PAGE 5: (In 1992, 43% of reproductive-age women expected to have an abortion) Henshaw SK. Unintended pregnancy in the United States. *Family Planning Perspectives.* 1998;30:24–29, 46. (In 2008, 30% of reproductive-age women expected to have an abortion) Jones RK, Kavanaugh ML. Changes in abortion rates between 2000 and 2008 and lifetime incidence of abortion. *Obstetrics & Gynecology*. 2011;117(6):1358–1366. (In 2014, 24% of reproductive-age women expected to have an abortion) Rachel K. Jones, Ph.D., Principal Research Scientist, Guttmacher Institute, personal communication, March 2017, based on a forthcoming article by Rachel K. Jones and Jenna Jerman.

PAGE 7: (the cases we discuss most are the ones that occur least) Girls 14 and under are 0.2% of abortion patients, and girls 15–17 are 3%. Jerman J, Jones RK, Onda T. *Characteristics of U.S. Abortion Patients in 2014 and Changes Since 2008* (Guttmacher Institute, 2016). In Guttmacher's 2014 survey of abortion patients, 1.4% said the pregnancy was a result of forced sex, and an additional 1.1% responded "don't know." These results will be published shortly after this book goes to press. Researchers don't currently collect data on how many abortions are for fetal anomalies, but Guttmacher's Principal Research Scientist informally estimates that's 1–2% of U.S. abortions. Rachel K. Jones, personal communication, November 2016. "Late abortion" is a minority as well. This is harder to quantify, because abortion is legal from conception to viability, which happens around 24 weeks. So what qualifies as a "late" abortion? Only 1.3% of abortions occur at 21 weeks or later. "Induced Abortion in the United States: January 2017 Fact Sheet," Guttmacher Institute. The "partial birth abortion" controversy revolved around the federal ban of an abortion procedure physicians typically called intact dilation and extraction (as opposed to "regular" or "traditional" D&E). There were no comprehensive statistics indicating what percentage of all abortions were performed in this manner, but researchers at the Guttmacher Institute estimated that in 2000, intact D&E procedures accounted for less than 1% of all abortions in the United States, approximately 0.17%. Finer LB, Henshaw SK. Abortion incidence and services in the United States in 2000. *Perspectives on Sexual and Reproductive Health.* 2003;35:6–15. Whether one calls an abortion done because the pregnancy threatens the woman's health "extraordinary" might depend on the severity of the condition. The most severe health threats are typically highlighted, but it's hard to define or quantify these. Finally, new debates about research on and disposal of fetal remains involve a larger number, but a minority of American abortion cases produce "fetal" remains. Before the end of the 10th week since a pregnant woman's last period, the entity aborted is an embryo. In Guttmacher's 2014 survey of abortion patients, researchers estimate that 81% of nonhospital abortions were performed at or before 10 weeks LMP. These results will be published shortly after this book goes to press. (Rachel K. Jones, personal communication, November 2016.)

Chapter 1

A NOTE ON ABORTION RESEARCH: In this chapter, my main source of data on the frequency of abortion and the characteristics of abortion patients is the Guttmacher Institute, a non-for-profit dedicated to reproductive research. No data are perfect, but on this topic, Guttmacher's are the best. The other primary source of abortion data is the Centers for Disease Control and Prevention (CDC), a federal agency. States are not required to report their abortion data to the CDC, but most do. Forty-six states require abortion providers to report their data, but statistics from these states vary in their completeness. And each state asks providers different questions, which makes national tallies impossible in some areas—for example, only 15 states require information about the woman's reason. In contrast, since 1974 Guttmacher researchers have reached out to all known abortion providers in the country (almost 2,000, including private physicians and hospitals that only perform a few each year) for annual surveys using standardized questions, plus new areas of research interest each year.

To maximize response rate, Guttmacher pursues extensive follow-up efforts for facilities that don't respond. For those that never respond, Guttmacher projects numbers—for example, of the 1.21 million abortions reported for 2005, 76% were reported by providers; 12% came from health department data; 9% were estimated by knowledgeable sources in the communities of the nonresponding clinics; and 3% were projections or other estimates. Guttmacher states that despite these efforts, past surveys of random samples of physicians and hospitals suggest that the true number of abortions is 3–4% greater than the number its reports estimate. "Abortion Reporting Requirements as of March 1 2015," Guttmacher Institute, State Policies in Brief. G. Sedgh and S. Henshaw, "Chapter 2: Measuring the Incidence of Abortion in Countries with Liberal Laws." In: S. Singh, L. Remez, and A. Tartaglione, eds. *Methodologies for Estimating Abortion Incidence and Abortion-Related Morbidity: A Review* (Guttmacher Institute and International Union for the Scientific Study of Population, 2010), 26–27. Finally, unlike the CDC, Guttmacher also periodically surveys patients as they are seeking abortions on topics like their reasons, religion, relationship status, and experiences with stigma.

Some claim Guttmacher data aren't reliable because the Institute is "pro-abortion." In contrast, I think Guttmacher's commitment to legal abortion and its prior relationship with Planned Parenthood increase, rather than decrease, the reliability of its research. Abortion providers are embattled, and it seems unlikely to me they would waste time voluntarily answering surveys from an organization they did not trust to be fair to them or their patients.

PAGE 17: (19% of pregnancies end in induced abortion) "Facts on Induced Abortion In the United States: January 2017," Guttmacher Institute, https://www.guttmacher.org/fact-sheet/induced-abortion-united-states [accessed Mar. 31, 2017].

PAGE 18: (Guttmacher abortion statistics do not include miscarriage) Rachel K. Jones, Ph.D., Principal Research Scientist, Guttmacher Institute, personal communication, November 2016. Of pregnancies that the body is continuing to support, 19% are intentionally ended with abortion, and 81% are carried to delivery. "Facts on Induced Abortion in the United States: January 2017," Guttmacher Institute. This number isn't published in Guttmacher reports, but staff estimate that 18% of pregnancies end in miscarriage. Special tabulations based on the authors' analysis of unintended pregnancies in 2011 from Finer LB, Zolna MR. Declines in unintended pregnancy in the United States, 2008–2011, *New England Journal of Medicine*. 2016;374(9):843–852.

PAGE 19: (the prevalence paradox) Kumar A, Hessini L, Mitchell EMH. Conceptualising abortion stigma. *Culture, Health & Sexuality: An International Journal for Research, Intervention, and Care*. 2009;11(6):625–639.

PAGE 19: The total number of abortions is higher than the number of individuals who have had abortions. This is because some women have more than one. The total number of abortions is reported, but the number of individual women who have had abortions since *Roe* is not typically reported. The number of individual women I use in this chapter was calculated for me in 2014 and conveyed through private communication by Stanley Henshaw, Ph.D., a sociologist who collected and analyzed abortion data while working at the Guttmacher Institute for decades. (He was a Senior Research Associate from 1979–1985, Deputy Director of Research 1985–1999, and Senior Fellow 2000–2013, and he is currently an independent consultant. I am grateful to Dr. Henshaw for an early review in 2014 confirming the numbers I used in that draft of this chapter were the most accurate available.) His data analysis leads him to conclude 28.4 million different women had legal abortions 1973–2010, and he estimates at least 500,000 had a first abortion each year from 2011 through 2014, for a total of 30.4 million first abortions 1973–2014.

PAGE 20: (reasons women have abortions) Finer LB, Frohwirth LF, Dauphinee LA, Singh S, Moore AM. Reasons U.S. women have abortions: quantitative and qualitative perspectives. *Perspectives on Sexual and Reproductive Health.* 2005; 37(3):110–118. Note this survey is more than 10 years old. I rely on it because it is the most recent research of its kind on women's reasons for having abortions, and the numbers reported are consistent with an earlier survey. In addition, Guttmacher has no current plans to do an updated version. Rachel K. Jones, personal communication, November 2016.

PAGE 20: (55 million abortions 1973–2014) Guttmacher staff estimate that 55,542,000 abortions occurred between 1973 and 2014. Rachel K. Jones, personal communication, July 2017.

PAGES 21, 31: (average U.S. woman has 1.8 children) 2015 fertility rates—World Bank, "Fertility Rate, Total (Births per Woman)," http://data.worldbank.org/indicator/SP.DYN.TFRT.IN?locations=US&view=chart [accessed June 10, 2017]. When data only analyzes women in the United States with children, the average number of children per mother goes up to 2.4. In 2014, 41% of American mothers had two children. Gretchen Livingston, "Family Size among Mothers." Pew Research Center, May 7, 2015. http://www.pewsocialtrends.org/2015/05/07/family-size-among-mothers/ [accessed June 10, 2017].

PAGE 23: (rape, incest, and me) E.g., Sella S. Maternal indications. *Atrium.* 2010;8:1–3 at 2 ("Unlike some anti-abortion patients who believe in abortion only in cases of rape, incest, and me"), http://www.bioethics.northwestern.edu/docs/atrium/atrium-issue8.pdf [accessed Mar. 31, 2017].

PAGE 23: "Scott DesJarlais supported ex-wife's abortions, slept with patients, divorce transcript shows: documents reveal liaisons with three coworkers, two patients and a drug rep." *Chattanooga Times Free Press,* Nov. 15, 2012, by Chris Carroll and Kate Belz, http://www.timesfreepress.com/news/news/story/2012/nov/15/scott-desjarlais-supported-abortions-slept-patient/92972/. "Tennessee GOP standing by congressman who compelled mistress to have abortion." *Times News,* Oct. 11, 2012, by Lucas L. Johnson, http://www.timesnews.net/article/9052818/tennessee-gop-standing-by-congressman-who-compelled-mistress-to-have-abortion.

PAGE 24: http://www.scottdesjarlais.com/issues/ [accessed Mar. 31, 2017].

PAGE 24: Congressman DesJarlais says he changed his beliefs over time. "DesJarlais said he is not the same man who supported his first wife's decision to have two abortions. . . . 'I guess as a physician, I was a fairly objective person,' he said of his beliefs at the time. 'I try not to be a judgmental person. [Abortion] was just not something that I put as much thought into as I should have, in retrospect. Going back, if I could change and do things differently, certainly I would.' " "DesJarlais: regret past actions, no plans to resign." *Knoxville News Sentinel*, Nov. 22, 2012, by Michael Collins, http://www.knoxnews.com/news/desjarlais-regret-past-actions-no-plans-to. Others have charged him with hypocrisy. "Which is more maddening—the absurd positions that right-wing Republicans take on abortion and other social issues, or the fact that they are so often shown to be complete hypocrites?" "Family values." *New York Times Editorial Page Editor's Blog*, Nov. 15, 2012, by Andrew Rosenthal, http://takingnote.blogs.nytimes.com/2012/11/15/family-values/?_r=0.

PAGE 24: (fundamental attribution error) Lee, "The Intuitive Psychologist and His Shortcomings: Distortions in the Attribution Process." In: L. Berkowitz, ed., *Advances in Experimental Social Psychology*, Volume 10 (Academic Press, 1977), 173–220.

PAGE 28: (58% of abortion patients say they need to keep it a secret) Shellenberg KM, Tsui AO. Correlates of perceived and internalized stigma among abortion patients in the United States: an exploration by race and Hispanic ethnicity. *International Journal of Gynecology and Obstetrics.* 2012;118(suppl 2):S152–S159.

PAGE 30: Approximately 233,000 new cases of breast cancer are diagnosed each year in the United States. Approximately 12% of American women will receive the diagnosis at some point in their lives. "SEER Stat Fact Sheets: Breast Cancer," National Cancer Institute, http://seer.cancer.gov/statfacts/html/breast.html [accessed Mar. 22, 2015].

PAGE 30: (45% of pregnancies are unintended, and 42% of those end in abortion) Finer and Zolna, Declines in unintended pregnancy. The category of unintended pregnancies includes those researchers call "mistimed" (with women who didn't want to become pregnant at the time it occurred, but did want to at some point in the future) and those researchers call "unwanted" (with women who did not want to become pregnant then or at anytime in the future). An earlier study analyzing the number of unintended pregnancies in 2008 reported that 31% of all pregnancies in the study were "mistimed" and 20% of all pregnancies were "unwanted." (These numbers add up to 2008's higher unintended pregnancy rate of 51%.) "Unintended Pregnancy in the United States: December 2013," Guttmacher Institute Fact Sheet.

PAGE 30: (89% find birth control morally acceptable) Art Swift, "Birth Control, Divorce Top List of Morally Acceptable Issues." Gallup Poll, June 8, 2016, http://www.gallup.com/poll/192404/birth-control-divorce-top-list-morally-acceptable-issues.aspx [accessed Mar. 31, 2017].

PAGE 31: (1800 fertility rates) Michael Haines, "Fertility and mortality in the United States." In: Robert Whaples, ed. *EH.Net Encyclopedia*, Mar. 19, 2008, http://eh.net/encyclopedia/fertility-and-mortality-in-the-united-states/ [accessed Mar. 17, 2015].

PAGE 31: (average age of U.S. women's first intercourse is 17) Centers for Disease Control and Prevention, National Center for Health Statistics, "National Survey of Family Growth 2011–2013," https://www.cdc.gov/nchs/nsfg/key-statistics/s.htm#vaginalsexual.

PAGE 31: (natural fertility rate—up to 29 abortions) Susan Harlap, Kathryn Kost, and Jacqueline Darroch Forrest, *Preventing Pregnancy, Protecting Health: A New Look at Contraception Choices in the United States* (Guttmacher Institute, 1991), 38 and Table 5.5. NOTE: This book says that if a fertile woman relies only on abortion and has no children, she will have 35 abortions over her lifetime. This equals an average of approximately 1.2 abortions per year. However, I say "up to 29 abortions" for two reasons. (1) The original calculation assumes fertility starts around age 15. However, I am proposing a hypothetical woman who starts having intercourse at 17, since that's the national average, and taking these two years off the sexually active fertility period reduces the estimated number of abortions needed by 2.4. (2) The original calculation assumes no children. I assume this hypothetical woman intends to have the national average of two births. These pregnancies and periods of breast feeding take approximately 3.35 years off of her fertile period, reducing the number of abortions by another 4. Similarly, another Guttmacher publication states, "Researchers have estimated that if a woman was continuously sexually active, did not use contraceptives and did not want any children, she would need to have more than 30 abortions in her lifetime." Jones RK, Singh S, Finer LB, Frohwirth LF. Repeat abortion in the United States. *Occasional Report No. 29*, November 2006, https://www.guttmacher.org/sites/default/files/report_pdf/or29.pdf [accessed Nov. 22, 2016].

PAGE 32: Trussell J. Contraceptive failure in the United States. *Contraception*. May 2011;83(5):397–404. This report reviews and summarizes multiple studies to create a comparison table intended to help patients understand the gap between perfect use and typical use when they pick a contraceptive. Note that the estimate of 85 pregnancies per 100 couples per year if using no form of contraception includes some number of people who would be naturally infertile. For a terrifying tabulation of the cumulative failure rate over 10 years of typical use, see "How Likely Is It That Birth Control Could Let You Down?" *New York Times,* Sept. 13, 2014, by Gregor Aisch and Bill Marsh (Condoms—86 pregnancies in 100 couples over 10 years; diaphragm—72 pregnancies in 100 couples over 10 years; pill/patch/ring—61 pregnancies in 100 couples over 10 years), http://www.nytimes.com/interactive/2014/09/14/sunday-review/unplanned-pregnancies.html?_r=0.

PAGE 32: (relationship between unintended pregnancy and contraceptive use) Dreweke J. New clarity for the U.S. abortion debate: a steep drop in unintended pregnancy is driving recent abortion declines. *Guttmacher Policy Review*. 2016;19:16–22, https://www.guttmacher.org/sites/default/files/article_files/gpr1901916.pdf [accessed Mar. 31, 2017].

PAGES 32–33: Leslie Jamison, *The Empathy Exams* (Graywolf Press, 2014), 18.

PAGE 33: (approximately one million illegal abortions per year) Gold RB. Lessons from before *Roe*: will past be prologue? *Guttmacher Report on Public Policy*, March 2003;6(1). Abortion rates between 1973 and 2014: Henshaw SK. Abortion Incidence and Services in the United States, 1995–1996. *Family Planning Perspectives*. 1998;30(6):263–270, 287. Jones RK, Jerman J. Abortion incidence and service availability in the United States, 2011. *Perspectives on Sexual and Reproductive Health*. 2014;46(1):3–14. Jones RK, Jerman J. Abortion incidence and service availability in the United States, 2014. *Perspectives on Sexual and Reproductive Health*. 2017;49(1):17–27.

PAGE 33: (In 1992, 43% of reproductive-age women expected to have an abortion) Henshaw SK. Unintended pregnancy in the United States. *Family Planning Perspectives*. 1998;30:24–29, 46. (In 2008, 30% of reproductive-age women expected to have an abortion) Jones RK, Kavanaugh ML. Changes in abortion rates between 2000 and 2008 and lifetime incidence of abortion. *Obstetrics and Gynecology*. 2011;117(6):1358–1366. (In 2014, 24% of reproductive-age women expected to have an abortion) Rachel K. Jones, Ph.D., Principal Research Scientist, Guttmacher Institute, personal communication, March 2017, based on a forthcoming article by Rachel K. Jones and Jenna Jerman.

PAGE 33: (researchers attribute lowered rates of unintentional pregnancy to contraception) Finer and Zolna, Declines in unintended pregnancy. See also Dreweke J. New clarity for the U.S. abortion debate: a steep drop in unintended pregnancy is driving recent abortion declines. *Guttmacher Policy Review*. 2016;19:16–22, https://www.guttmacher.org/sites/default/files/article_files/gpr1901916.pdf [accessed Mar. 31, 2017].

PAGE 34: Sociologist Kristen Luker made the helpful analogy to other types of health-risk behaviors in her groundbreaking book decades ago, and many aspects of it still ring true today. Kristin Luker, *Abortion and the Politics of Motherhood* (University of California Press, 1985).

Chapter 2

PAGES 39–40: H. Porter Abbott, *The Cambridge Introduction to Narrative*, 2nd ed. (Cambridge University Press, 2008), 179. ("[A] trial can be described as … the contest of two sets of authors, each trying to make their central narrative of events prevail by spinning narrative segments for their rhetorical impact.")

For more on masterplots, see Abbott at 46–49, 185, and 236 ("National culture is a complex weave of numerous, often conflicting, masterplots." 48). It's also interesting to note that masterplots "often come equipped with types—characters whose motivation and personality are an integral and often fixed element of the masterplot." (185) For more on overreading and underreading narratives, see Abbott at 239 and pages noted therein. For more on counter-narratives, see Abbott at 188.

PAGE 40: Lawyers are well trained in the idea of constructing a case and the power of the question that frames the case. However, a book that deepened my thinking in this area comes from bioethics. In *The Fiction of Bioethics* (Routledge, 1999) my colleague Tod Chambers set aside the content of ethics case presentations, all of which contained only true facts, and instead analyzed them as narratives, identifying fundamental elements of their construction such as character, narration, and plot, and examining how choices in case framing helped to justify ethical conclusions.

PAGE 41: *Roe v. Wade*, 410 U.S. 113 (1973). For more facts about the life of "Jane Roe" (and the other players, and the drama of how *Roe v. Wade* unfolded in the courtroom), see Peter Irons, *The Courage of Their Convictions: Sixteen Americans Who Fought Their Way to the Supreme Court* (Penguin Books, 1988). Norma McCorvey (the real "Jane Roe") died shortly before this book went to press. For an insightful tribute about the complexity of her life, see Loretta Ross, "Mourning Norma McCorvey," https://bitchmedia.org/article/mourning-norma-mccorvey/story-jane-roe-lifelong-struggle-heal-hardship-and-abuse [accessed Mar. 25, 2017].

PAGE 42: In *The Fiction of Bioethics,* Chambers also points out how bioethicists have used a medical style of case presentation, covertly adopting a physician voice perhaps to adopt physicians' authority. (27) It is fair to argue Justice Blackmun was doing something similar in *Roe.*

PAGE 42: Justice White's dissent to *Roe* appears at the end of *Doe v. Bolton,* 410 U.S. 179, 221–223 (1973), and an asterisk footnote on the first page of Justice White's dissent says "This opinion applies also to No. 70-18, *Roe v. Wade,* ante, p. 113." *Doe* was a companion case to *Roe* in which the Court elaborated on the scope of *Roe*'s exception allowing abortion after viability for women's life and health. Justice Rehnquist also wrote his own short dissent in *Roe,* but it focused exclusively on procedural and constitutional questions without telling any particular "abortion story."

PAGE 43: *Planned Parenthood of Southeastern Pa. v. Casey,* 505 U.S. 833 (1992).

PAGE 45: (patient right to refuse medical treatment) E.g., *Cruzan v. Director, Mo. Dep't of Health,* 497 U.S. 261 (1990).

PAGE 46: An account of the negotiations that led to the *Casey* majority and minority opinions can be found in Jeffrey Toobin, *The Nine: Inside the Secret World of the Supreme Court* (Anchor Books, 2008).

PAGE 47: *Gonzales v. Carhart*, 550 U.S. 124 (2007).

PAGE 47: ACOG stated that the 2007 Supreme Court decision on "partial birth abortion" "discounts and disregards the medical consensus that intact D&E is safest and offers significant benefits for women suffering from certain conditions that make the potential complications of non-intact D&E especially dangerous." http://www.acog.org/About-ACOG/News-Room/News-Releases/2007/ACOG-Statement-on-the-US-Supreme-Court-Decision [accessed Apr. 3, 2015].

PAGE 47: The Court drew the quote from the nurse who "witnessed" the procedure from her testimony before the Senate Judiciary Committee. She says the procedure she saw was done on a 26-week fetus. Because that's after the usual line for viability, it is likely this abortion was done to preserve the life or health of the pregnant woman, or because the fetus had severe anomalies. In *The Fiction of Bioethics*, Chambers points out the narrative significance of direct quotes ("reported discourse"): in bioethics cases they mark moments of high drama (118, 126). It's not common to see direct quotes from witnesses in appellate court opinions, and reading Chambers made me realize the same is true in the majority opinion of *Carhart*.

PAGE 48: The *Carhart* decision devotes significant space to medical details. It's easy to overlook the fact that getting a fetus or baby out of a woman's body is violent however it happens. In my twenties I volunteered at a public hospital to be a doula (a coach for women in labor) for low-income women without partners or family in the delivery room. I did this because I believe in reproductive justice (the ability to both have, and not have, babies) and delivering alone sounded like a hard way to start motherhood for women who didn't want that. But I almost fainted the first time I saw a baby explode out of a woman's body. The blood, the screams, the smells, the ripping ... intellectually I knew it was a good thing, but the videos and readings I absorbed in training couldn't prepare me for the visceral violence of it. The same was true the first time a woman I accompanied in childbirth required a caesarian section. The top part of her body was happily chatting away, but on the other side of the blue drape (which she asked me to watch and narrate) they cut her open with what looked like a straight razor. A bloody baby was extracted from her abdominal cavity and her sliced uterus was set outside her body like a piece of offal until it could be stitched up. Again, intellectually I was perfectly aware she was under local anesthesia and this was a safe and good thing. But at a visceral level everything in me was screaming, "They're gutting this lady! Call the police!" After a few deliveries my brain and heart synched up, and I experienced both forms of delivery as natural. Similarly, I predict that at first it would be hard for me to watch a second-trimester abortion (whether intact or not), and that after watching a few abortions that might also become normalized. Vaginal delivery, caesarian delivery, and abortion have different outcomes. What they have in common is that each is what the pregnant woman or couple thought was the right thing to do, and that like most medical procedures, they all are likely to feel somewhat gruesome to people outside of medicine.

PAGE 49: The *Carhart* majority's claim of severe depression and loss of esteem following abortion may be true for some, but the American Psychological Association and American Psychiatric Association have both concluded abortion is not harmful to mental health. Many studies have shown abortion does not cause depression, and in many cases, it improves emotional states. For a summary and list of many of these studies, see David A. Grimes, with Linda G. Brandon, *Every Third Woman in America: How Legal Abortion Transformed Our Nation* (Daymark, 2014), 197–213.

PAGE 50: ("difficult decision" masterplot) Writer Katha Pollitt has noticed this framing as well: "How often have you heard abortion described as 'the hardest decision' or 'the most painful choice' a woman ever makes, as if every single woman who gets pregnant by accident seriously considers having a baby, only a few weeks earlier the furthest thing from her mind and for a very good reason. Or more accurately, as if every accidentally pregnant woman really *should* seriously consider having that baby—and if she doesn't at least claim that she thought long and hard about it and only reluctantly and sadly realized it was impossible, she's a bad woman who thinks only of her own pleasure and convenience." She also cites two examples of commentators opining on how women "ought" to feel, both published in *The New Republic*: "In a much-reprinted 1995 essay, Naomi Wolf . . . urged women who ended their pregnancies to feel guilt and to mourn their fetuses" and Andrew Sullivan "thinks 'abortion is always and everywhere a moral tragedy.' " Katha Pollitt, *Pro: Reclaiming Abortion Rights* (Picador, 2014), 30, 37.

PAGE 51: Steinbock B. Why abortion decisions are not always difficult. *Atrium*. 2008;5:22, http://www.bioethics.northwestern.edu/about/atrium/ [accessed Apr. 3, 2017].

PAGE 53: (abortion regret) Watson K. Reframing regret. *JAMA*. 2014;311(1):27–28. Kimport K. (Mis)understanding abortion regret. *Symbolic Interaction*. 2012;35(2):105–122.

PAGE 53: Rocca CH, Kimport K, Roberts SCM, Gould H, Neuhaus J, Foster DG. Decision rightness and emotional responses to abortion in the United States: a longitudinal study. *PLoS ONE*. 10(7):e0128832. doi:10.1372/journal.pone.0128832.

PAGE 55: (the dignity of risk) Perske R. The dignity of risk and the mentally retarded. *Mental Retardation*. 1972;10(1):24–27; Parsons C. The dignity of risk: challenges in moving on. *Australian Nursing Journal*. 2008;15(9):28; Mukherjee D. Discharge decisions and the dignity of risk. *The Hastings Center Report*. 2015;45(3):7–8.

PAGE 58: Leslie Jamison, *The Empathy Exams* (Graywolf Press, 2014), 1–26.

PAGE 59: Willie Parker, *Life's Work: a Moral Argument for Choice* (Atria Books, 2017), 144–145.

PAGE 60: (88% of abortion patients are married or dating) In this study 12% report they are not in a relationship; here I am reporting the opposite implication of that number. Jones RK, Finer LB, Singh S. *Characteristics of U.S. Abortion Patients, 2008.* (Guttmacher Institute, May 2010), Figure 1. https://www.guttmacher.org/report/characteristics-us-abortion-patients-2008 [accessed June 2017].

PAGE 61: (male knowledge and support of abortion) Jones RK, Moore AM, Frohwirth LH. Perceptions of male knowledge and support among U.S. women obtaining abortions. *Women's Health Issues.* 2011;21(2):117–123. Women who had been exposed to intimate partner violence by the man with whom they became pregnant (physical abuse or forced to do something sexual) were significantly less likely to report he knew about the abortion (62%, vs. 84% of the women with no IPV).

PAGE 68: (44% in dating relationship) This number is my deduction—in the study cited above, 12% of women having abortions say they are not in a relationship, 15% are married, and 29% are cohabiting. That totals 56%, leaving 44% as saying they are in a relationship which doesn't involving living with their parenter (married or cohabiting), which I have described as "dating." Jones et al., *Characteristics of U.S. Abortion Patients, 2008* (Guttmacher Institute, 2010). In 2014, two of these numbers changed slightly—14% of abortion patients were married and 31% cohabitating—but this study did not document how many were in other romantic relationships or the length of relationships, so I used the earlier numbers. Jerman J, Jones RK, Onda T. *Characteristics of U.S. Abortion Patients in 2014 and Changes Since 2008* (Guttmacher Institute, 2016), https://www.guttmacher.org/report/characteristics-us-abortion-patients-2014.

PAGE 68: (relationship length over and under one year) Jones et al., *Characteristics of U.S. Abortion Patients, 2008* (Guttmacher Institute, 2016).

PAGE 68: (59% of abortion patients are already mothers) Jerman J, Jones RK, Onda T. *Characteristics of U.S. Abortion Patients in 2014.* See also Jones RK, Frohwirth LF, Moore AM. "I would want to give my child, llike, everything in the world": how issues of motherhood influence women who have abortions. *Journal of Family Issues.* 2008;29(1):79–99.

PAGE 70: Sabine Roeser, *Moral Emotions and Intuitions* (Springer, 2010).

PAGE 71: *Bowers v. Hardwick,* 478 U.S. 186 (1986) (upholding Georgia statute criminalizing sodomy).

PAGES 71, 72: *Lawrence v. Texas,* 539 U.S. 558 (2003) (striking Texas statute criminalizing same-sex sex).

PAGE 72: For an excellent analysis of how the model of gay people coming out is relevant to abortion rights, see Skinner-Thompson S, Law SA, Baran H. Marriage, abortion and coming out. *Columbia Law Review Online.* 2016;116:126–151.

PAGE 74: Harris LH, Martin L, Debbink M, Hassinger J. Physicians, abortion provision and the legitimacy paradox. *Contraception*. 2013;87:11–16.

Chapter 3

PAGE 79: (case of Aaron Harrison) *State v. Harrison*, 2011 UT 74 (Utah 2011).

PAGES 80, 81, 82: *Roe v. Wade*, 410 U.S. 113 (1973). The *Roe* decision's terminology for what a pregnant woman carries varies greatly, perhaps because it was written before each term got so loaded. Terms used in *Roe* include: the unborn, her pregnancy, potential life, prenatal life, embryo, fetus, potential human life, when life begins, unborn children, and the potentiality of human life.

PAGE 83: E.g., Scheper-Hughes, N. Culture, scarcity, and maternal thinking: maternal detachment and infant survival in a Brazilian shantytown. *Ethos*. 1985;13:291–317. This anthropologist studied 72 poor women 17–71 years old (median age 39) living in a context of high child mortality. On average the women in this shantytown sample delivered 8 live babies, 3–4 of whom died before age 5 (70% before 6 months old). "Many Alto babies remain not only unchristened but *unnamed* until they begin to walk or talk... ." [In healthy children, first steps usually occur between 9–12 months, and first words around 12 months.] Sadly, "[p]art of learning how to mother on the Alto includes learning when to 'let go.'" Scheper-Hughes's research leads her to argue "that maternal thinking and practices are socially produced rather than determined by a psychobiological script of innate or universal emotions... ." She contrasts the historically recent and culturally specific Western reproductive strategy of giving birth to few babies and investing heavily in each one with a high expectation of survival, with the different approach of giving birth to many children, investing selectively, and hoping a few survive—a "reproductive strategy [that] requires a very different conception of maternal thinking, and just as surely elicits different kinds of maternal attachments, feelings, and sentiments. ... Since this reproductive strategy is characteristic of much of the world's poorer population today, it would seem that some revision of maternal bonding/maternal thinking as a universal human script is in order." In the Brazilian context she studied, child funerals were an almost daily occurrence, and "'[m]otherlove'... is replaced by an estranged and guarded 'watchful waiting.' What makes this possible is a cultural conception of the child as human, but significantly less human than the grown child or adult."

PAGE 85: Howard Rheingold asserts that the apocryphal saying is Eskimos have 17 words for snow. But "the real action in the Eskimo language is in the category of 'ice,'" for which Rheingold asserts they have 170 words. Howard Rheingold, *They Have a Word for It: A Lighthearted Lexicon of Untranslatable Words and Phrases* (Jeremy P. Tarcher, 1988), 208–210. (Reprinted in 2000 by Sarabande Books.)

PAGE 86: (80% of abortions occur before 10 weeks LMP; 8 weeks conception) "Fact Sheet: Induced Abortion in the United States," Guttmacher Institute, January 2017, https://www.guttmacher.org/fact-sheet/induced-abortion-united-states#2 [accessed Apr. 2, 2017].

PAGE 87: *State v. J.M.S*, 2011 UT 75 (Utah 2011). The prosecution of pregnant women is a critical issue that is beyond the scope of this book. A rich source of current information on the topic is National Advocates for Pregnant Women, www.advocatesforpregnantwomen.org. For a bioethics analysis of some of these issues, see Bonnie Steinbock, *Life Before Birth: The Moral and Legal Satus of Embryos and Fetuses*, 2nd ed. (Oxford University Press, 2011), Section 4, "Maternal-Fetal Conflict."

PAGE 88: Utah Code 76-5-201. (This criminal homicide law states it does not apply to women having abortions with physicians, or those who refuse caesarian sections or other medical care knowing it could lead to fetal demise.)

PAGE 88: Erich Goode and Nachman Ben-Yehuda, *Moral Panics: The Social Construction of Deviance* (Blackwell, 1994); Kenneth Thompson, *Moral Panics* (Routledge, 1998); Stanley Cohen, *Folk Devils and Moral Panics* (MacGibbon and Kee, 1972).

PAGE 89: (details on J.M.S.'s personal circumstances) "Policing Pregnancy." *The Nation.* May 9, 2011, by Michelle Goldberg; "Utah teen may face criminal charges in abortion beating case." *Salt Lake Tribune*, Dec. 14, 2011, by Melinda Rogers; "Utah Supreme Court: Teenager who paid for assault in hope of abortion liable." *Deseret News* (Utah), Dec. 13, 2011, by Emiley Morgan.

PAGE 90: (ten Utah teens get pregnant each day) According to The National Campaign to Prevent Teen and Unplanned Pregnancy, 3,530 15- 19-year-old women in Utah got pregnant in 2011. (2,163 of these pregnancies resulted in births.) https://thenationalcampaign.org/data/state/utah. If that total were divided evenly across the 365 days of the year, it would be 9.67 pregnancies per day.

PAGE 90: (72-hour wait for abortion) Utah Code 76-7-305.

PAGE 90: (10-week abortion costs approximately $500) Jerman J, Jones RK. Secondary measures of access to abortion services in the United States, 2011 and 2012: gestational age limits, cost, and harassment. *Women's Health Issues.* 2014;24(4):e419–e424.

PAGE 91: (written consent of a parent or guardian required for Utah minor abortion) Utah Code 76-7-304.5.

PAGE 91: (Utah restrictions on sex ed) Utah public school health classes are prohibited from adopting materials that include "the advocacy or encouragement of the use of contraceptive methods or devices." Utah Code 53A-13-101-1(c) iii(A)III. See also Rose Aguilar, "Utah Governor Signs Controversial Law Charging Women and Girls with Murder for Miscarriages," Alternet.org, Mar. 8, 2010 [accessed Feb. 4, 2015].

PAGES 91–92: Loretta J. Ross and Ricki Solinger, *Reproductive Justice: An Introduction* (University of California Press, 2017).

PAGE 95: (number of abortions happening in the second trimester) "Fact Sheet: Induced Abortion in the United States," Guttmacher Institute, January 2017.

PAGE 96: (In 2000, intact D&E procedures accounted for approximately 0.17% of all abortions in the U.S.) Finer, Henshaw. Abortion incidence and services in the United States in 2000. *Perspectives on Sexual and Reproductive Health.* 2003;35:6–15.

PAGE 96: *Stenberg v. Carhart,* 530 U.S. 914 (2000).

PAGE 96: Partial-Birth Abortion Ban Act of 2003, 18 U.S.C. §1531; Congressional findings on the Act, Pub. L. 108–105, §2, Nov. 5, 2003, 117 Stat. 1201.

PAGE 96: *Gonzales v. Carhart,* 550 U.S. 124 (2007).

PAGE 96: (three elements of moral panic) Cohen, *Folk Devils,* "Chapter 2: The Inventory."

PAGE 97: The article below contains a link to the full Gallup survey, which reports the details of the survey. Gallup asked "With respect to the abortion issue, would you consider yourself to be pro-choice or pro-life?" and 3% volunteered the answer "Mixed/neither." So of course the framing of the question may have steered some people away from answering with more nuance. (50% picked pro-choice, 44% picked pro-life, 2% volunteered that they didn't know what the terms meant, and 1% said they had no opinion.) Lydia Saad, "Americans Choose 'Pro-Choice' for first time in seven years," *Gallup Social Issues,* May 29, 2015, http://www.gallup.com/poll/183434/americans-choose-pro-choice-first-time-seven-years.aspx [accessed Apr. 2, 2017]. Gallup's article on its 2016 survey does not include a link to the detailed information, but since it reports similar numbers (47% pro-choice, 46% pro-life, totaling 93% with a position as compared to 94% reporting a position in 2015), it's fair to assume there hasn't been a radical jump in those reporting a mixed position. Lydia Saad, "Americans' Attitudes toward abortion unchanged." *Gallup Social Issues,* May 25, 2016, http://www.gallup.com/poll/191834/americans-attitudes-toward-abortion-unchanged.aspx [accessed Apr. 2, 2017].

Chapter 4

PAGE 99: According to a sign accompanying the embryonic and fetal specimens at the Museum of Science and Industry, they were collected in the 1930s by Dr. Helen Button of Loyola Medical Center and Michael Reese Hospital: "To the best of our knowledge, all failed to survive because of accidents or natural causes. Dr. Button obtained the parents' permission to use these specimens as teaching tools." To the Museum's credit, it's added something to its collection of embryos and fetuses that wasn't there in my childhood—now a new kiosk describing changes in a pregnant woman's body greets you at the exhibit's entrance.

PAGE 99: (What if women's cadavers were displayed?) In fifth grade my mom gave me an awesome Christmas present—an educational toy called the Visible Woman that allowed you to assemble tiny plastic organs and a tiny plastic skeleton and click them into place inside a 16-inch woman made of clear plastic. The part that fascinated me most was the "Optional Feature: The Miracle of Creation." If you wanted the Visible Woman to be seven months pregnant, you assembled a separate set of parts, clicking a tiny plastic fetus into a uterus, replacing her small intestines with a version that draped around that uterus, and replacing her clear chest plate with one contoured for a see-through pregnancy. I didn't remember Ms. VW when I was at the museum, but writing about my alternate exhibit fantasy made me remember how I loved clicking her pregnancy in and out. If unconscious memory of her is what made me think pregnancy only makes sense seen in the context of a pregnant woman, perhaps her educational mission was a success. http://americanhistory.si.edu/collections/search/object/nmah_214318.

PAGE 100: (optical illusion) "My wife and my mother-in-law." W.E. Hill, *Puck*, November 6, 1915 (adapted from an earlier drawing). "I'MMORAL" does something similar linguistically—in a poster advertising a fundraiser for California Planned Parenthood, an apostrophe flips the meaning of the word emblazoned across a woman's body. Milton Glaser and Mirko Ilić, *The Design of Dissent* (Rockport, 2005), 115.

PAGE 101: (pluralism defense of abortion) See also Watson K. The unacknowledged consensus on abortion. *American Journal of Bioethics*. 2010;10(12):57–59.

PAGE 102: (Some argue that if we're uncertain about the moral status of embryos and fetuses, we should err on the side of not destroying them) E.g., Tomasz Zuradzki describes this argument before using it to analyze whether embryo research is morally permissible. (Of course, when an embryo resides in a lab instead of in a woman and she has donated it for research, the lack of her countervailing interest might tip the scales of uncertainty about embryos differently.) Zuradzki T. Moral uncertainty in bioethical argumentation: a new understanding of the pro-life view on early human embryos. *Theoretical Medicine and Bioethics*. 2014;35:441–457. David Boonin critiques the argument in his book, *A Defense of Abortion* (Cambridge University Press, 2003). A summary of Boonin's critique and a response to it defending the precautionary principle can be found in Friberg-Fernros H. Taking precautionary concerns seriously: a defense of a misused antiabortion argument. *Journal of Medicine and Philosophy*. 2014;39(3):228–247.

PAGE 105: (89% of abortions occur before 12 weeks LMP; 66% before 8 weeks LMP) "Fact Sheet: Induced Abortion in the United States," Guttmacher Institute, January 2017, https://www.guttmacher.org/fact-sheet/induced-abortion-united-states#2 [accessed Apr. 2, 2017].

PAGE 106: (38% of Catholics say abortion is morally acceptable) Jeffrey M. Jones, "US Religious Groups Disagree on Five Key Moral Issues," Gallup Social Issues, May 26, 2016, http://www.gallup.com/poll/191903/religious-groups-disagree-five-key-moral-issues.aspx [accessed Apr. 5, 2017]. (24% of abortion patients report they are Roman Catholic) Jerman J, Jones RK, Onda T. *Characteristics of U.S. Abortion Patients in 2014 and Changes Since 2008* (Guttmacher Institute, 2016), https://www.guttmacher.org/report/characteristics-us-abortion-patients-2014 [accessed Apr. 5, 2017].

PAGE 107: (Substantial Identity Theory) E.g., Lee P. The pro-life argument from substantial identity: a defence. *Bioethics*. 2004;18(3):249–263. Beckwith FJ. The explanatory power of the substance view of persons. *Christian Bioethics*. 2004;10.1:33–54.

PAGE 107: (Potential Theory) Marquis further explores and defends his "future like ours" argument in multiple publications, but his original description of it can be found here: Marquis D. Why abortion is immoral. *Journal of Philosophy*. 1989;86(4):183–202. See also Engelhardt Jr, HT. The ontology of abortion. *Ethics*. 1974;84(3):217–234. Wade FC. Potentiality in the abortion discussion. *Review of Metaphysics*. 1975;239–255. Parness JA, Pritchard SK. To be or not to be: protecting the unborn's potentiality of life. *University of Cincinnati Law Review*. 1982;51:257.

PAGE 108: (Critiques of substantial identity and potentiality theory) E.g., Katha Pollitt, *Pro: Reclaiming Abortion Rights* (Picador, 2015), 69, 96–97, 57; Reiman J. The pro-life argument from substantial identity and the pro-choice argument from asymmetric value: a reply to Patrick Lee. *Bioethics*. 2017;21(6):329–341.

PAGE 110: (definition of autonomy) Tom L. Beauchamp and James F. Childress, *Principles of Biomedical Ethics*, 7th ed. (Oxford University Press, 2012). The first edition of this book was published in 1977, and the ideas it contained had an enormous impact on the newly developing field of bioethics. In the forty years that have followed, many more philosophical approaches to bioethics have emerged, but the fact many are reactions against, or amendments to, the principlist framework speaks to its continuing influence.

PAGE 111: Ann Furedi, *The Moral Case for Abortion* (Palgrave McMillan, 2017), 80.

PAGE 112: Thomson JJ. A defense of abortion. *Philosophy and Public Affairs*. 1971;1(1):47–66.

PAGE 113: *McFall v. Shimp,* 10 Pa. D. & C. 3d 90 (1978). One could argue that transplant isn't analogous because in pregnancy, nine months later you get your organs back. A refined analogy might point to living-donor kidney transplant (after which donors live well with just one kidney), or living-donor liver transplant (in which the donor gives a liver lobe and the body regenerates that piece in a few months). The promise of recovery doesn't lead us to force those either.

PAGE 114: For more analysis of the analogy between lethal self-defense and what the author calls "medical self-defense" in the context of abortion, the right of the terminally ill, and payment for organs, see Volokh E. Medical self-defense, prohibited experimental therapies, and payment for organs. *Harvard Law Review.* 2007;120(7):1813–1846.

PAGE 114: (slavery analogy) Some who oppose abortion compare themselves to abolitionists trying to save fetuses who are like slaves. As Debora Threedy points out, "both sides of the abortion debate have appropriated the image of the slave and used that image as a rhetorical tool, a metaphor, in making legal arguments." Threedy D. Slavery rhetoric and the abortion debate. *Michigan Journal of Gender and Law.* 1994;3(2):3–25. One law professor has argued that the prohibition against slavery in the U.S. Constitution could and should provide alternate grounds for a constitutional right to abortion. But one doesn't have to be persuaded by this legal argument to be persuaded by this ethical argument. Koppelman A. Originalism, abortion, and the Thirteenth Amendment. *Columbia Law Review.* 2012;112:1917.

PAGES 114–115: Willie Parker, *Life's Work: A Moral Argument for Choice* (Atria Books, 2017), 107–108.

PAGE 116: (adoption) Before 1973, about 9% of infants overall and 20% of infants born to white never-married women were relinquished. Between 1996 and 2002, only 1% of babies born to never-married women were relinquished. Jones J. Who adopts? Characteristics of women and men who have adopted children. *NCHS Data Brief.* January 2009;12, https://www.cdc.gov/nchs/data/databriefs/db12.pdf [accessed Apr. 9, 2017]. (adoption by women turned away from abortion facilities). Sisson G, Ralph L, Gould H, Greene Foster D. Adoption decision making among women seeking abortion. *Women's Health Issues.* 2017;27(2):136–144.

PAGE 116: (The Veil of Ignorance.) John Rawls, *A Theory of Justice* (Belknap Press, 1971). Rawls uses the Veil of Ignorance as an exercise to establish the "original position," the organizing institutions and set of constitutional principles that form the foundation of society. In later works he details his idea of "public reason" (which he sometimes calls "reasonable pluralism")—arguments that appeal to reason, fairness, and civility—as a way to select specific social policies for that society, and he names abortion as an example of a contentious issue that secular reasoning focused on equality would conclude should be legal. John Rawls, *Political Liberalism: Expanded Edition* (Columbia University Press, [1993] 2005); John Rawls, *Justice as Fairness,* 2nd ed. (Belknap Press, 2001).

PAGE 117: (Some argue the Veil of Ignorance approach shows that abortion is unjust.) E.g., John Finnis argues that Rawls's protection of children as "future citizens" means he should logically extend this protection to fetuses. John Finnis, "Abortion, Natural Law, and Public Reason." In: R. P. George and C. Wolfe, eds. *Natural Law and Public Reason* (Georgetown University Press, 2000), 75–106.

PAGE 120: The "responsibility critique" of Jarvis Thomson's argument is widespread. For example, these writers argue all her argument proves is the permissibility of abortion after rape: Robert Wennberg, *Life in the Balance: Exploring the Abortion Controversy* (William B. Eerdman, 1985); Paul Feinberg, "The Morality of Abortion." In: Richard L. Ganz, ed. *Thou Shalt Not Kill: The Christian Case against Abortion.* (Arlington House, 1978), 127–149. For a response, see Boonin-Vail D. A defense of "A Defense of Abortion": on the responsibility objection to Thomson's argument. *Ethics.* 1997;107(2):286–313, 298. ("[A] person's act cannot be taken as tacitly consenting to anything unless it takes place in a context where it is generally understood as constituting such consent.")

PAGE 123: (relationship between unintended pregnancy and contraceptive use) Dreweke J. New clarity for the U.S. abortion debate: a steep drop in unintended pregnancy is driving recent abortion declines. *Guttmacher Policy Review.* 2016;19:16–22, https://www.guttmacher.org/sites/default/files/article_files/gpr1901916.pdf [accessed Mar. 31, 2017].

PAGES 125–129: (Public Health Ethics) Lawrence O. Gostin, ed., *Public Health Law and Ethics*, 2nd ed. (University of California Press, 2010); Baron H. Lerner and Ronald Bayer, "History of Public Health Ethics in the United States." In: Robert B. Baker and Laurence B. McCullough, eds., *Cambridge World History of Medical Ethics* (Cambridge University Press, 2009), 655–666.

PAGE 126: David A. Grimes with Linda G. Brandon, *Every Third Woman in America: How Legal Abortion Transformed Our Nation* (Daymark, 2014).

PAGE 130: Personal communication with Lynn Paltrow April 7, 2017, confirming comments she made during Q&A while a panelist at a NAF conference.

PAGE 130: (Care ethics) Carol Gilligan, *In a Different Voice: Psychological Theory and Women's Development* (Harvard University Press, 1982); Nel Noddings, *Caring: A Feminine Approach to Ethics and Moral Education* (University of California Press, 1984). See also "Care Ethics," by Maureen Sander-Staudt, *The Internet Encyclopedia of Philosophy*, http://www.iep.utm.edu/care-eth/.

PAGE 131: Susan Sherwin, *No Longer Patient: Feminist Ethics and Health Care* (Temple University Press, 1992).

PAGE 132: Callhan S. Abortion and the sexual agenda: a case for pro-life feminism. *Commonweal.* Apr. 25, 1986;232. Reprinted in: Robert M. Baird and Stuart E. Rosenbaum, eds. *The Ethics of Abortion: Pro-Life vs. Pro-Choice*, 3rd ed. (Prometheus Books, 2001).

PAGE 134: Bonnie Steinbock, *Life before Birth: The Moral and Legal Status of Embryos and Fetuses*, 2nd Ed. (Oxford University Press, 2011), 81.

PAGES 135–139: Mary Anne Warren, *Moral Status: Obligations to Persons and Other Living Things* (Clarendon Press, 1997). Philosophers like John Rawls and Peter Singer offer general accounts of moral status as well.

PAGE 140: (45% of abortion patients in 2014 have had one previously) Jones RK, Jerman J, Ingerick M. Which abortion patients have had a prior abortion? Findings from the 2014 U.S. Abortion Patient Survey. *Journal of Women's Health,* forthcoming. This is a decrease—in 2008 50% of abortion patients had one previously. (Interestingly, in 2008 37% of patients had a history of both prior birth and prior abortion.) Jones RK, Finer LB, Singh S. *Characteristics of U.S. Abortion Patients, 2008* (Guttmacher Institute, May 2010), Figure 2. https://www.guttmacher.org/report/characteristics-us-abortion-patients-2008 [accessed June 2017].

PAGE 140: (ethical underpinning of Roe and Casey) As Beauchamp and Childress point out, "Legal decisions often express communal moral norms." However, the authors add, "[n]o body of abstract moral principles and rules can fix policy in such circumstances [of disagreement]. The implementation of moral principles and rules must take into account factors such as feasibility and efficiency, cultural pluralism... . Principles and rules provide the moral background for policy formation and evaluation, but policy must also be shaped by empirical data... ." "The judgment that an act is morally wrong does not necessarily lead to the judgment that the government should prohibit it or refuse to allocate fund to support it. For example, one can argue without inconsistency, that sterilization and abortion are morally wrong but the law should not prohibit them, because they are fundamentally matters of personal choice beyond the authority of the government (or, alternatively because many persons would seek dangerous and unsanitary procedures from unlicensed practitioners)." Tom L. Beauchamp, James F. Childress, *Principles of Biomedical Ethics*, 7th ed. (Oxford, 2012).

PAGE 143: Little MO. Abortion and the margins of personhood. *Rutgers Law Journal*. 2008;39:331, 341.

Chapter 5

Unless otherwise noted, in this chapter all description of embryological and fetal attributes and identification of what week in gestation (by conception dating) each developmental stage occurs is from Larry R. Cochard, *Netter's Atlas of Embryology*, updated ed. (Elsevier, 2012), and all statistics about when abortion occurs are from "Induced Abortion in the United States: Fact Sheet, January 2017," Guttmacher Institute. https://www.guttmacher.org/fact-sheet/induced-abortion-united-states [accessed Mar. 5, 2017].

PAGE 145: (Scientism) Caplan A, Marino TA., The role of scientists in the beginning-of-life debate: A 25-year retrospective. *Perspectives in Biology and Medicine*. 2007;50(4):603–613, 609.

PAGE 150: (LMP dating) American Congress of Obstetricians and Gynecologists. Method for estimating due date. Committee Opinion No. 611. *Obstetrics and Gynecology*. 2014;124:863–866.

PAGES 151–152: (EC not abortifacient) "What an abortifacient is—and isn't." *National Catholic Reporter*, Feb. 20, 2012, by Jamie Mason, https://www.ncronline.

org/blogs/grace-margins/what-abortifacient-and-what-it-isnt. See also "Facts Are Important: Emergency Contraception (EC) and Intrauterine Devices (IUDs) Are Not Abortifacients," American Congress of Obstetricians and Gynecologists, June 12, 2014, http://www.acog.org/-/media/Departments/Government-Relations-and-Outreach/FactsAreImportantEC.pdf?dmc=1 [accessed Apr. 10, 2017].

PAGE 152: *Burwell v. Hobby Lobby,* 573 U.S. ____ , 134 S. Ct. 2751 (2014).

PAGE 152: (only 8 states allow EC without a prescription) Guttmacher Institute. "Emergency Contraception." Apr. 1, 2017, https://www.guttmacher.org/state-policy/explore/emergency-contraception [accessed Apr. 10, 2017].

PAGE 153: (ensoulment cannot happen until fourteen days after conception) E.g, Cahill LS. The embryo and the fetus: new moral contexts. *Theological Studies.* 1993;54(1):124–142.

PAGE 153: (ART—men have equal say in how to use frozen embryos) E.g., *Davis v. Davis,* 842 S.W.2d 588, 597 (Tenn. 1992). But see *Szafranski v. Dunston,* 2015 IL App 1st 122975 B, *cert. denied,* 136 S. Ct. 1230 (2015) (Boyfriend of woman about to undergo egg-destroying cancer treatments gave his sperm knowing this was her "last chance to preserve her fertility." Since she could have used an anonymous sperm donor to preserve her opportunity to have a genetically related child, when they broke up and he changed his mind, the court treated her reliance on his promise as an exception to the general rule allowing male veto.)

PAGE 154: (North Dakota ban on abortion after fetal heartbeat) N.D. Cent. Code §14-02.1. Courts later ruled it was unconstitutional: *MKB Mgmt. Corp. v. Stenehjem,* 795 F.3d 768 (8th Cir. 2015), *cert. denied,* 136 S. Ct. 981 (2016). In 2016 at least five other state legislatures considered heartbeat bans: Alabama, Indiana, New York, Ohio, and South Carolina.

PAGE 155: (shift from embryo to fetus) Faces are hard for medical students too. Anatomy class requires those studying medicine to dissect a dead human adult. Most future doctors can summon the detachment necessary to focus on their anatomy lessons while they dissect, but many students report that cutting the face and the hands are emotionally difficult. Looking at these parts, it's impossible to forget their cadaver used to be a person.

PAGE 157: Mifeprex REMS Study Group. Sixteen years of overregulation: time to unburden Mifeprex. *New England Journal of Medicine.* 2017;376(8):790–794.

PAGE 158: (quickening) According to the Supreme Court in the *Roe* decision, at common law (the law English judges made over centuries of accumulated case decisions that those in the American colonies inherited and adapted to make their own), abortion was not a crime if performed before quickening. In 1821 Connecticut was the first state to enact abortion legislation prohibiting abortion for a woman "quick with child." In 1828, New York made destruction of a quickened fetus second-degree manslaughter, and destruction of an unquickened fetus a misdemeanor. Many states followed New York's model in the following century, until the 1950s, when "a large majority of the jurisdictions banned abortion, however and whenever performed, unless done to save or preserve the life of the mother."

PAGE 160: (neonatal mortality and morbidity) Stoll BJ, et al. Trends in care practices, morbidity, and mortality of extremely preterm neonates, 1993–2012. *JAMA*. 2015;314(10):1039–1051. The National Institute of Child Health and Human Development has a calculator that allows people to learn about neonatal survival odds based on several factors, https://www.nichd.nih.gov/about/org/der/branches/ppb/programs/epbo/pages/epbo_case.aspx [accessed Apr. 11, 2017].

PAGE 161: (the viability paradox) Watson K. Abortion bans premised on fetal pain capacity. *Hastings Center Report*. 2012;42(5):10–11.

PAGES 162–163: (18 states have "fetal pain" bans) "State Policies on Later Abortions," Guttmacher Institute, June 1, 2017, https://www.guttmacher.org/state-policy/explore/state-policies-later-abortions [accessed June 15, 2017].

PAGE 163: (cases striking 20-week pain bans as unconstitutional) *Isaacson, M.D. v. Horne*, 716 F.3d 1213, 1217 (9th Cir. 2013)—Arizona; *McCormack v. Herzog*, 788 F.3d 1017 (9th Cir. 2015)—Idaho.

PAGES 163–164: (scientific consensus is fetal pain happens at or after 26 weeks) Lee SJ, Ralston HJ, Drey EA, Patridge JC, Rosen MA. Fetal pain: a systematic multidisciplinary review of the evidence. *JAMA*. 2005;294(8):947–954. Royal College of Obstetricians and Gynecologists, *Fetal Awareness: Review of Research and Recommendations for Practice* (March 2010), https://www.rcog.org.uk/globalassets/documents/guidelines/rcogfetalawarenesswpr0610.pdf [accessed Dec. 8, 2016]. "Facts Are Important: Fetal Pain," ACOG, July 2013, https://www.acog.org/-/media/Departments/Government-Relations-and-Outreach/FactAreImportFetalPain.pdf [accessed Dec. 8, 2016].

PAGE 164: Peter Singer, *Practical Ethics*, 2nd ed. (Cambridge University Press, 1997), 166.

PAGE 165: "State Policies on Later Abortions," Guttmacher Institute, June 1 2017.

PAGE 165: (organized cortical activity) David Boonin, *A Defense of Abortion* (Cambridge University Press, 2003). See also Vanhatalo S, Kaila K. Development of neonatal EEG activity: from phenomenology to physiology. *Seminars in Fetal & Neonatal Medicine*. 2006;11:471–478.

PAGE 166: (brain death criteria) Uniform Determination of Death Act, http://www.uniformlaws.org/shared/docs/determination%20of%20death/udda80.pdf [accessed Apr. 10, 2017]; Eelco FM, et al. Evidence-based guideline update: determining brain death in adults. *Neurology*. 2010;74:1911–1918.

PAGE 172: Katha Pollitt, *Pro: Reclaiming Abortion Rights* (Picador, 2015), 11.

PAGE 174: (42% of 2.8 million unintended pregnancies end in abortion) Finer LB, Zolna MR. Declines in unintended pregnancy in the United States, 2008–2011. *New England Journal of Medicine*. 2016;374:843–852.

Chapter 6

PAGE 176: (being attentive to power is part of a bioethicist's job) Howard Brody, *The Healer's Power* (Yale University, 1992).

PAGE 176: (Trojan Horse laws) After developing this analysis, it was affirming to learn others have viewed these laws this way as well. E.g., Siegel S, Blustain S. Mommy dearest. *The American Prospect.* 2006:22–26 at 26 ("With anti-abortion drafting and incremental litigation strategies, the informed-consent paradigm could turn out to be the Trojan horse that will take down *Roe.*"); Jordan B, Wells ES. A 21st-century Trojan horse: the "abortion harms women" anti-choice argument disguises a harmful movement. *Contraception.* 2009;79(3):161–164.

PAGE 176: (10 times more likely to die of colonoscopy) *Whole Woman's Health v. Hellerstedt,* 579 US ___, 136 S. Ct. 2292 (2016) at 2315.

PAGE 176: (admitting privileges conditioned on a certain number of admissions per year) *Whole Woman's Health,* at 2312.

PAGES 177, 178: *Whole Woman's Health v. Lakey,* 46 F.Supp. 3d 673, 681, 684 (2014); *Whole Woman's Health v. Cole,* 790 F.3d 563, 576, 584, 587 (per curiam), *modified,* 790 F.3d 598 (CA5 2015); *Whole Woman's Health v. Hellerstedt,* at 2310.

PAGE 179: Johanna Schoen, *Abortion after Roe* (University of North Carolina Press, 2015).

PAGE 179: (protests rose in 1980s) Schoen, *Abortion,* 170–174; 187–188.

PAGE 179: (siege of Wichita) Willie Parker, *Life's Work: A Moral Argument for Choice* (Atria Books, 2017), 124.

PAGE 180: (protests declined in the 1990s) Schoen, *Abortion,* 188, 194, 196.

PAGE 180: (intense protests turned patients away) Schoen, *Abortion,* 193, 175.

PAGE 180: "U.S. Marshals Dispatched to Guard Abortion Clinics." *The Washington Post,* August 2, 1994, by Pierre Thomas, https://www.washingtonpost.com/archive/politics/1994/08/02/us-marshals-dispatched-to-guard-abortion-clinics/80067334-dd30-4a0a-9a00-bfa438da968a/?utm_term=.9c79961431d4. *See also,* Department of Justice, National Task Force on Violence Against Health Care Providers. https://www.justice.gov/crt/national-task-force-violence-against-health-care-providers-0

PAGES 180, 181: (flood of abortion laws) "Laws Affecting Reproductive Health and Rights: 2014 State Policy Review," Guttmacher Institute, https://www.guttmacher.org/laws-affecting-reproductive-health-and-rights-2014-state-policy-review; "Policy Trends in the States: 2016" Guttmacher Institute, https://www.guttmacher.org/article/2017/01/policy-trends-states-2016 [accessed Mar. 22, 2017].

PAGE 182: (29 states dictate "informed consent" content) Thirty-five states have abortion-specific informed consent laws; 6 of them generally follow the established principles of informed consent and 29 of them detail the information a woman must be given. "Counseling and Waiting Periods for Abortion as of

March 1, 2017," Guttmacher Institute, https://www.guttmacher.org/state-policy/explore/counseling-and-waiting-periods-abortion [accessed Mar. 22, 2017].

PAGE 182: (26 states regulate ultrasound) "Requirements for Ultrasound as of March 1, 2017," Guttmacher Institute, https://www.guttmacher.org/state-policy/explore/requirements-ultrasound [accessed Mar. 22, 2017]. *See also* Weitz T, Kimport K. The discursive production of abortion stigma in the Texas ultrasound viewing law. *Berkeley Journal of Gender Law & Justice*. 2015; 30:6-21.

PAGE 183: (27 states have waiting periods) "Counseling and Waiting Periods for Abortion as of March 1, 2017," Guttmacher Institute. See also "Waiting Periods for Abortion," Guttmacher Institute, February 2017, https://www.guttmacher.org/evidence-you-can-use/waiting-periods-abortion [accessed Mar. 22, 2017].

PAGE 184: (original concept of stigma) Erving Goffman, *Stigma: Notes on the Management of Spoiled Identity* (Simon & Schuster, 1963).

PAGE 184: Link BG, Phelan J. Stigma power. *Social Science & Medicine*. 2014;103: 24–32. See also Hatzenbuehler ML, Link BG. Introduction to the special issue on structural stigma and health. *Social Science & Medicine*. 2014;103:1–6.

PAGES 184–185, 197–198: (race analogy) Other authors have noted the parallel between racial and reproductive discrimination. The authors of *Crow After* Roe point to how legal attacks on the abortion right after *Roe* have segregated abortion clinics from mainstream medicine, and argue that "[a]s the federal courts had done with slavery and Jim Crow laws in the nineteenth century, *Casey* established a two-tier system of those who had access to the basic trappings of citizenship, and those who did not." Robin Marty and Jessica Mason Pieklo, *Crow After* Roe*: How "Separate But Equal" Has Become the New Standard in Women's Health* (Brooklyn, NY: Ig, 2013), 15. Lynn Paltrow calls fetal personhood bills and the incarceration of pregnant women they inspire "The New Jane Crow." Paltrow LM. *Roe v. Wade* and the New Jane Crow: Reproductive rights in the age of mass incarceration. *American Journal of Public Health*. 2013;103(1):17–21. I understand that some fetal rights advocates see this analogy in reverse: they say our era's version of racism is seeing an embryo or fetus as less than a full person, and those who advocate for embryonic or fetal rights are like civil rights leaders who worked to change laws discriminating against people of color.

PAGE 186: (92% have mind made up before making abortion appointment) Moore AM, Frohwirth L, Blades N. What women want from abortion counseling in the United States: A qualitative study of abortion patients in 2008. *Social Work in Health Care*. 2011;50(6):424–442.

PAGES 186–187: Alissa C. Perrucci, *Decision Assessment and Counseling in Abortion Care: Philosophy and Practice* (Rowman and Littlefield, 2012), 19.

PAGE 187: (risk of death in childbirth is approximately 14 times higher than in abortion) Raymond EG, Grimes DA. The comparative safety of legal induced abortion and childbirth in the United States. *Obstetrics & Gynecology*.

2012;119:215–219. (up to 1 in 7 get postpartum depression). "Postpartum Depression," American Psychological Association, http://www.apa.org/pi/women/resources/reports/postpartum-depression.aspx [accessed June 18, 2017].

PAGE 187: (waiting periods) Legislators who refuse to trust the intelligence of adult patients and the integrity of physicians and counselors should turn what's already "best practice" in medical counseling into law—prohibit *any* patient getting *any* medical procedure who isn't sure about their medical choice and would benefit from a delay from receiving their medical procedure that day, be it gallbladder removal, chemotherapy, or abortion. If a bill like this were introduced (whether by a fair-minded anti-abortion legislator, or a pro-choice legislator amending an abortion-only waiting period), a lack of interest would confirm that abortion-only waiting periods aren't meant to support patient decision-making, they're meant to impose stigma and obstacles on abortion alone.

PAGE 189: Lori Freedman, *Willing and Unable: Doctors' Constraints in Abortion Care* (Vanderbilt University Press, 2010), 18, 15, 99, 103, 111. Freedman interviewed thirty ob/gyns. Some were prevented from providing abortion care because they worked in religiously affiliated healthcare facilities, and some were in private practices but could not (except for the one) find a way to provide abortions. The number of subjects in each category is not specified in Freedman's book, and because some subjects had worked in multiple settings over the years, might be hard to identify exactly.

PAGE 189: (only half of residents who intended to provide abortions did so) Steinauer J, Landy U, Filippone H, Laube D, Darney PD, Jackson RA. Predictors of abortion provision among practicing obstetrician-gynecologists: a national survey. *American Journal of Obstetrics & Gynecology*. 2008;198:39.e1–39.e6. This study surveyed 2,149 ob/gyns who finished residency between 1990 and 1998, and were board certified between 1998 and 2001. Despite the fact many finished training before 1996, when the requirement that all ob/gyn residency programs provide abortion training (with opt-out choices) took effect, 73% went to residency programs where abortion training was available. Interestingly, 5% who did not intend to provide abortions before residency, and 19% who were uncertain, ended up doing so. "Providing abortion" was defined as doing an elective abortion within the last year.

PAGE 190: Consistent with Freedman's observation about child care, 72% of the ob/gyns providing abortions had children, according to the survey by Steinauer et al. Freedman also points out how the trend toward group practice, and the policies that allow one doctor opposed to abortion to control the group's policy, particularly affects obstetricians with young children. It's better for parents to join large groups, because higher numbers of providers reduce the number of nights they have to take overnight call. But large groups have higher odds one person in the group will oppose abortion. Freedman, *Willing and Unable*, 15–16.

PAGE 193: Why does Midwestern Hospital only do "medically indicated" abortions and not "elective" abortions? "Because it's [State]?" the ethicist ventured. "Some of it has to do with avoiding public embarrassment. Because there are regular pickets at Planned Parenthood where the procedure happens."

PAGE 196: (extremists turned to violence) Schoen, *Abortion,* 197.

PAGE 196: (11 murdered) "A brief history of deadly attacks on abortion providers." *New York Times,* Nov. 29, 2015, by Liam Stack, https://www.nytimes.com/interactive/2015/11/29/us/30abortion-clinic-violence.html. For analysis of the link between violence and the public identification and vilification of doctors who provide abortion, see "Who killed George Tiller." *The Guardian,* June 1, 2009, by Jill Filipovic, https://www.theguardian.com/commentisfree/cifamerica/2009/jun/01/george-tiller-abortion-doctor-murder. In 1997 an anti-abortion activist created a website called "The Nuremberg Files" that listed the names and addresses of doctors who provided abortions, including Barnett Slepian. A different man killed Dr. Slepian in his home in front of his wife and children 1998. In 2002, Operation Rescue (now called Operation Save America) moved its headquarters to Kansas to focus on Dr. George Tiller, maintaining a "Tiller Watch" website that listed his whereabouts. In 2009, a man who did not belong to Operation Rescue shot and killed Dr. Tiller at his church. In 2015, a few months after surreptitiously filmed Planned Parenthood videos were put on the internet, a man who did not belong to the group that made the videos went on a shooting spree at a Planned Parenthood in Colorado Springs, reportedly saying "no more baby parts" to the police after the shooting. "Abortion witch hunt." *New York Times,* Mar. 4, 2016, by Amanda Robb. There may be additional murders and violent attacks driven by the same goals. "The terrorist campaign against abortion." *Village Voice,* Nov. 10, 1998, by Jennifer Gonnerman, http://www.villagevoice.com/news/the-terrorist-campaign-against-abortion-6423113.

PAGE 196: National Abortion Federation. *2015 Violence and Disruption Statistics* (April 2016), https://5aa1b2xfmfh2e2mk03kk8rsx-wpengine.netdna-ssl.com/wp-content/uploads/2015-NAF-Violence-Disruption-Stats.pdf [accessed Apr. 10, 2017].

PAGE 199: "Fact Sheet: Women in the US Congress 2017," Center for American Women and Politics (CAWP), Eagleton Institute of Politics, Rutgers University, 2015, http://www.cawp.rutgers.edu/women-us-congress-2017 [accessed Apr. 12, 2017].

PAGE 200: *Bradwell v. State of Ill.,* 83 U.S. (16 Wall.) 130 (1872).

PAGE 200: (number of women law students and lawyers) Brief of amici curiae Janice Macavoy et al., submitted Jan. 4, 2016, in *Whole Woman's Health v. Cole,* and sources cited therein, at 13, http://www.scotusblog.com/wp-content/uploads/2016/01/Janice-Macavoy-Paul-Weiss.pdf [accessed Apr. 10, 2017].

PAGE 201: Law SA. Rethinking sex and the Constitution. *University of Pennsylvania Law Review.* 1984;132:955. http://scholarship.law.upenn.edu/

cgi/viewcontent.cgi?article=4602&context=penn_law_review; Ginsburg RB. Some thoughts on autonomy and equality in relation to *Roe v. Wade. North Carolina Law Review.* 1985;63:375. (William T. Joyner Lecture, University of North Carolina School of Law, Apr. 6, 1984), http://scholarship.law.unc.edu/nclr/vol63/iss2/4.

PAGE 201: E.g., Siegel RB. The new politics of abortion: an equality analysis of woman-protective abortion restrictions. *University of Illinois Law Review.* 2007:991-1054; Siegel RB. The right's reasons: constitutional conflict and the spread of woman-protective antiabortion argument. *Duke Law Journal.* 2008;57:1641–1692; Siegel RB. Dignity and the politics of protection: abortion restrictions under *Casey/Carhart. Yale Law Journal.* 2008;117:1694–1800.

PAGES 202, 204: Ioannes Paulus PP. II, *Evangelium Vitae* (Mar. 25, 1995), http://w2.vatican.va/content/john-paul-ii/en/encyclicals/documents/hf_jp-ii_enc_25031995_evangelium-vitae.html [accessed Aug. 24, 2016].

PAGE 203: *Griswold v. Connecticut,* 381 U.S. 479 (1965).

PAGE 203: *Eisenstadt v. Baird,* 405 U.S. 438 (1972).

PAGE 204: *Carey v. Population Services,* 341 U.S. 68 (1977).

PAGE 206: Link and Phelan, Stigma power, 31.

PAGE 207: (income status of abortion patients) Jerman J, Jones RK, Onda, T. *Characteristics of U.S. Abortion Patients in 2014 and Changes Since 2008* (Guttmacher Institute, 2016), https://www.guttmacher.org/report/characteristics-%20us-abortion-patients-2014 [accessed Apr. 12, 2017].

PAGE 207: "2014 Poverty Guidelines," U.S. Department of Health and Human Services, https://aspe.hhs.gov/2014-poverty-guidelines [accessed Apr. 10, 2017].

PAGES 208–209: (rates of unintended pregnancy and abortion by income) Finer LB, Zolna MR. Declines in unintended pregnancy in the United States, 2008–2011. *New England Journal of Medicine.* 2016;374:843–852, Tables 1 and 2.

PAGE 209: (risk rises) E.g., F. Gary Cunningham, et al., eds. *Williams Obstetrics,* 24th ed. (McGraw-Hill Education, 2014), Ch. 18. ("Early abortions are even safer, and the relative mortality risk of abortion approximately doubles for each 2 weeks after 8 weeks' gestation.").

PAGES 217–218: Brief of amici curiae Macavoy et al., *Whole Women's Health v. Cole.*

Epilogue

PAGE 219: (professors don't talk about private lives) Of course there are exceptions. Anthropologist Rayna Rapp and philosopher Paul Lauritzen write that their personal experiences with prenatal testing and infertility treatment, respectively, inspired their scholarship in these areas. In contrast, my scholarly analysis of abortion largely preceded my intimate experience with the topic.

Reyna Rapp, *Testing Women, Testing the Fetus: The Social Impact of Amniocentesis in America* (Routledge, 2000); Lauritzen P. What price parenthood? *Hastings Center Report*. 1990;20(2):38–46. See also Lauritzen P. Ethics and experience: the case of the curious response. *Hastings Center Report*. 1996;26(1):6–15.

PAGE 220: "Shout Your Abortion" invites women to videotape themselves telling their abortion stories for viewing on YouTube, or to write about them on Twitter, to match "the volume of the opposition, but we shout about reality, not lies." "#ShoutYourAbortion is committed to changing culture, building community, and setting people on the path of freedom by telling the truth about abortion: Abortion is common, necessary, and supported by the majority of Americans." https://shoutyourabotion.com/about [accessed June 10, 2017]. Other storytelling projects include the 1 in 3 Campaign, and We Testify. http://www.1in3campaign.org/written-stories, https://wetestify.org/stories/.

PAGES 220, 221: (better story to think with) Here I'm inspired by sociologist's Charles Bosk's reflections on what an ethnographer chooses to include and exclude in order to preserve anonymity in the stories told from their fieldwork. "[T]hough veracity was a goal, though a commitment to getting the facts right was what separated ethnography from fiction, I still had told a good story, a useful story. … What was important was to create a version of reality that would in Levi-Strauss's memorable formula be 'good to think with.'" Charles Bosk, *Forgive and Remember: Managing Medical Failure*, 2nd ed. (University of Chicago Press, 2003), 216.

PAGE 223: (the clinic is better) The difference between the clinic's and hospital's methods that affected timing was how the cervix is dilated before the abortion. The clinic used misoprostol ("miso") pills that dissolve in your cheek over the course of two hours. The hospital inserted laminaria into the cervix, which causes it to dilate over the course of about a day. That's why the hospital method required patients to come in two days in a row.

PAGE 225: (paid out of pocket) In 2014, "most patients with private health insurance (61%) paid out of pocket for their abortion." Jerman J, Jones RK, Onda, T. *Characteristics of U.S. Abortion Patients in 2014 and Changes Since 2008* (Guttmacher Institute, 2016). Note that the number of patients who had private insurance coverage for abortion but did not use it could be lower than 61%, because this study did not follow up to confirm how many of the unused private insurance plans actually *covered* abortion. Another study found that 77% of abortion patients with private insurance "did not or could not use it to pay for their abortion," instead paying an average of $578. Roberts SCM, Gould H, Kimport K, Weitz TA, Greene Foster D. Out-of-Pocket Costs and Insurance Coverage for Abortion in the United States. *Women's Health Issues*. 2014;24(2):e211–e218.

PAGE 227: (the advantages of high-volume single-procedure clinics) Atul Gawande, *Complications* (Picador, 2002).

INDEX